ALSO FROM NONVELLA

Far From Home
VARIOUS AUTHORS

Foodville
TIMOTHY TAYLOR

The Silicon Rapture
ADAM PEZ

The Shoe Boy
DUNCAN McCUE

Where I'd Rather Go
VARIOUS AUTHORS

OPIUM EATER: THE NEW CONFESSIONS
Copyright © 2016 Nonvella Publishing Inc.

ALL RIGHTS RESERVED
No part of this publication may be reproduced, stored in a retrieval system or transmitted in any form or by any means, electronic, mechanical, photocopying, recording or otherwise, without permission obtained from Nonvella Publishing Inc. or the author.

www.nonvella.com

Cover illustration by Slavka Kolesar
Book design by Strand Design Studio
Edited by Tyee Bridge

Printed and bound in Canada

Library and Archives Canada Cataloguing in Publication:
Zwarenstein, Carlyn, author
    Opium eater : the new confessions / Carlyn Zwarenstein.

Includes bibliographical references.
Issued in print and electronic formats.
ISBN 978-0-9936216-8-0 (paperback).
—ISBN 978-0-9936216-9-7 (ebook)

1. Zwarenstein, Carlyn—Health. 2. Zwarenstein, Carlyn—Drug use. 3. Pain—Treatment. 4. Authors—Drug use. 5. Opium—Therapeutic use. 6. Opium abuse. 7. Opium abuse in literature. I. Title.

HV5805.Z83A3 2016   362.29092   C2016-901918-7
                                          C2016-901924-1

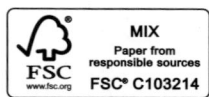

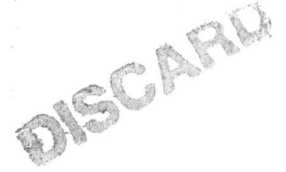

OPIUM EATER
The New Confessions

CARLYN ZWARENSTEIN

NONVELLA

For Etien and Theo, with love.
"IF NOT DUFFERS WON'T DROWN"

"If the entire materia medica at our disposal were limited to the choice and use of only one drug, I am sure that a great many, if not the majority, of us would choose opium; and I am convinced that if we were to select, say half a dozen of the most important drugs in the Pharmacopeia, we should all place opium in the first rank."

—Pharmacologist David I. Macht, writing in the Journal of the American Medical Association, 1915

Wynken, Blynken, and Nod one night
Sailed off in a wooden shoe—
Sailed on a river of crystal light,
Into a sea of dew.
"Where are you going, and what do you wish?"
The old moon asked the three.

TODAY I AM flying from Toronto to New York City. Travel—formerly my great delight—has lately become something of an ordeal. My neck cranes forward, pushed by stiff, hunching shoulders. The muscles at the front of my neck are as short and tight as steel cables; a dull burn at the back of my neck radiates down to my tailbone. My lower back feels unstable, an oddly unbearable sensation, as if my spinal column were inadequate to support the rest of me.

I have a spine disease called ankylosing spondylitis (AS). One of the particular torments of this condition is an inability to find comfort either sitting down or standing up. Seated in the departure lounge, I shift and wriggle in my seat.

I take a little pill bottle from the pocket of my coat and hold it in my hand.

Through the window, the water in the harbour is slate blue, the financial district buildings beside it are grey and blue as well, reflecting dull sky and dull water. It's like being in a black and white movie—or a cyanotype, rather, bluescale. What a November day. But I am going on holiday. I've left my loved ones at home for the weekend, and now, for the next six hours, I'm about to leave pain behind as well—along with its accompanying stress, sorrow, and existential angst.

I chase the pale yellow pill, an opioid called tramadol, with a bitter sip of coffee.

The radar weather on the TV screen above me shows a shifting, restless display of green-on-green clouds. It's a good metaphor for the feeling I have during the hour or so after the pill: all the weather in me churning and gathering up and clearing itself out. I'm calm but alert. Anticipating. I still feel the pain that dogs me, but already its force is provisional, its minutes numbered. It no longer depresses me as it so easily can do.

At last, with an unforced sigh as I'm released from pain, I finally lean back in my seat. The airport chatter is muted now. There is a faraway clattering of glasses, and the cackle of friends laughing off to my right is now more distant. A man in a blue surgical mask cleans white cups off a table. As I take in the details, I begin to notice my breath going in and out—my stomach slowly rising and falling, air sweeping through my nostrils, down the back of my throat, filling up my lungs. A seagull floats unsteadily on the rough breezes outside.

By the time my flight is called I'm able to stand up briskly, limber and quick. I walk carefully to my gate, smile serenely at the attendant as my passport and boarding pass are checked, and glide into the airplane. The sky has brightened, the cloud cover lifted.

As I settle into my seat, successive waves of good feeling wash over me like the surf. My holiday has begun.

IN HER BOOK *A Field Guide to Getting Lost*, Rebecca Solnit writes of opiates and their effect of turning her "into something almost reptilian."

"Opiates," she writes, turn you "into a cool spectator of your own sensations and desires and of passing time, as languorous as all those images of divans and draperies and long pipes had promised."

YES. FOR THE relief of severe pain, I take painkillers derived from and inspired by opium. I have taken morphine, extracted from the sap or resin of the opium poppy (and so an "opiate," a subset of the larger category, opioids); hydromorphone, a strong, semi-synthetic opioid made from morphine; and tramadol, a relatively weak synthetic opioid with a structure similar to codeine and morphine.

All three of these drugs temporarily mask symptoms of my condition, against which even unhealthy amounts of Tylenol don't stand a chance. They do so without the major side effects I've experienced with other medicines. Of the three, I like tramadol the best. It works on the brain both as an opioid and also somewhat like a Prozac-type antidepressant. Tramadol relieves pain incredibly well, helps me sleep through physical discomfort, and perks my mood enough to manage the demands of the day.

ANKYLOSING SPONDYLITIS IS a degenerative autoimmune disease. A form of inflammatory arthritis, it typically strikes young people in their prime—in my case, at twenty-eight, shortly after the first of my two sons was born. AS is roughly analogous to having rheumatoid arthritis in the spine. My immune system attacks my body, causing chronic inflammation that began in the sacroiliac joints at the base of the spine and for the past ten years has been gradually moving upward.

In his 2001 novel *Austerlitz*, the writer W.G. Sebald describes an ankylosing spondylitis patient:

> [...] lying down was perhaps even more painful for him than walking, so that as a rule, despite his exhausted state after his constant perambulations, it was a long time before he could get to sleep. Then, through the grille of a ventilation shaft [...] he could be heard calling on numerous different saints for hours on end, in particular, if I remember correctly, Saints Catherine and Elizabeth, who suffered the most cruel of martyrdoms, begging them to intercede for him in the contingency, as he put it, of his imminent appearance before the judgment seat of his Heavenly Lord.

It came out of the blue. The disease and resulting pain have devastated my life. I'm still trying to find my way now, a decade later.

In severe AS, inflammation causes the vertebrae to fuse together by a process of erosion and remodelling of the bone. If I'm unlucky, bone will form between my vertebrae and I will be left with a completely immobile, terribly fragile spinal column, or "bamboo spine." Two gut-shredding years of anti-inflammatory medicines left me with an ulcer, debilitating heartburn, and various food intolerances, as well as constant fear of potential side effects—like sudden and occasionally fatal gastrointestinal bleeding and heart attacks.

"I will never take those again," I told the rheumatologist, standing uncomfortably rather than sitting in the chair I'd been offered. The doctor wrote me a prescription and handed it over across his desk. It was only after googling "tramadol" that I learned I'd been prescribed my first opioid.

THE OPIUM POPPY has been cultivated for over three thousand years. The Sumerians called it *hul gil*, the joy plant. The nineteenth century—the

Romantic and early- to mid-Victorian period—was the great age of opium, with derivative medicines used by patients of all ages for all manner of ailments. Addiction at that time was viewed for the most part as a weakness rather than either a criminal act or a medical condition, and the opium trade itself was a cornerstone of British imperial policy.

Morphine—named for the god of sleep, dreams, and transformation—was first isolated from the sap of the poppy (that is, opium) by 1805 by a German pharmacist's apprentice. Friedrich Sertürner was also an opium addict, and later, not surprisingly, a morphine addict. Morphine is the most important active constituent of opium, and its isolation—along with the development of the hypodermic needle mid-century—allowed for more straightforward and effective pain management. In all cases, an injection makes the drug dramatically stronger and faster-acting, and more dangerous.

Morphine remains the gold standard drug against which all other opioids, including the synthetic ones, are compared, dosing of all of them being calculated in terms of equivalencies of morphine. Morphine and its derivatives are the most effective and powerful painkillers around today. While legal and prescribed for medical reasons, these substances are related to currently illegal drugs such as heroin—itself synthesized by an English chemist and once sold freely as a cough suppressant. (It works.)

While heroin was made illegal in the United States in 1925, in the late forties and fifties you could still pick up your prescription for heroin pills at the Boots pharmacy in Piccadilly Circus in London—in fact, under its medical name diamorphine, it is still used in the U.K. as a strong painkiller.

AS A GIRL, I loved the Sherlock Holmes stories, and read and reread Arthur Conan Doyle's erotically measured lines about the famous seven percent solution of cocaine:

> Sherlock Holmes took his bottle from the corner of the mantelpiece and his hypodermic syringe from its neat morocco case. With his long, white, nervous fingers he adjusted the delicate needle, and rolled back his left shirt-cuff. For some little time his eyes rested thoughtfully upon the sinewy forearm and wrist all dotted and scarred with innumerable puncture-marks. Finally he thrust the sharp

point home, pressed down the tiny piston, and sank back into the velvet-lined arm-chair with a long sigh of satisfaction.

Like him, I enjoy the waiting. Once I have decided that today is going to be a tramadol day, and I've given myself a deadline before which I absolutely will not cave in and take it, my experience of pain is transformed. Rather than grinding and hopeless, it feels charged, electric. The difficulty I have standing up (or sitting down) begins to feel noble. The constant, miserable, and exhausting stretching I do to relieve pain and stiffness in my joints acquires a warm-up quality.

I am already removed one degree from my own experience and it is a little more observable, a little more interesting. I know that in a little while, after some sore but delicious anticipation, it will melt away in an exquisitely gradual, perceptible way. And then I will feel expansive and happy. The hours ahead are no longer to be endured but rather to be savoured, and this knowledge invigorates me, refocusing my day.

Then there is the actual taking of the drug. If you don't get a high from whatever medicine *you* take, I suppose it is just a medicine. Nobody craves Tylenol or ibuprofen or Lipitor. If, however, the drug you are taking is really, in your own mind, a drug, all the preparation involved is part of a lovely ritual of anticipation. It has a sort of a pleasant glow of association. Do this, feel that. A lifelong non-smoker, a cautious adolescent, and the most sober adult at any party, I have nevertheless been fascinated by intoxication, addiction, and altered mental states for as long as I can remember.

I don't think that anyone I know has known that about me.

The flame that licks the spoon. The tightening of the rubber strap and the clinical flicking of a tube with the nails of index finger and thumb. The way you hold the cigarette, even, stretching out your fingers, touching your lips as you inhale. It's all a very private romance.

Unfortunately for my sense of occasion and aesthetics, all *I* do is swallow a medium-sized yellowish pill, chasing it with some water or—more sensibly, given the drowsiness it induces—coffee.

THE MOST NOTORIOUS drug addict in English letters was a man named Thomas De Quincey. He was born in 1785 and died in 1859. De Quincey was perhaps the best essayist in English in an age when creative non-fiction, as it's called today, was having its moment. He chronicled his vivid memories of the pain and pleasures of medicinal opium in his memoir, *Confessions of an English Opium-Eater*:

> Opium! Dread agent of unimaginable pleasure and pain! I had heard of it as I had of manna or of ambrosia, but no further. How unmeaning a sound was it at that time: what solemn chords does it now strike upon my heart! What heart-quaking vibrations of sad and happy remembrances! Reverting for a moment to these, I feel a mystic importance attached to the minutest circumstances connected with the place and the time and the man (if man he was) that first laid open to me the Paradise of Opium-eaters.

By *man-if-man-he-was* he means the pharmacist. (The humble apothecary is also described as the "beatific vision of an immortal druggist, sent down to earth on a special mission to myself.") In his *Confessions*, as he wrote in a revised edition late in life, De Quincey hoped to "emblazon the power of opium—not over bodily disease and pain, but over the grander and more shadowy world of dreams." Blurring the line between addiction and pleasure, recreational and medical use, he anticipated Freud in his exploration of the effect of the subconscious on the psyche.

De Quincey's father was a relatively prosperous merchant who died when De Quincey was a child. Two of his sisters also died when he was young. He was especially traumatized by the early death of his elder sister Elizabeth, probably of meningitis, and haunted by imagined visions—which returned during the nightmares of opium withdrawal in later life—of her skull, which he saw (or believed he'd seen) when it was opened for an autopsy.

As a teenager, De Quincey ran away from his much-hated Manchester boarding school and decamped to Wales and then London. He nearly starved to death in the big city before embarking on a career as an essayist and hack writer, churning out hundreds of essays for the leading publications of the day. A charming, eccentric, and sometimes pitiful man as an adult, De Quincey was ambitious, versatile, eloquent, and (as the number of exclamation points in the above excerpt suggest) often over-the-top as a writer. And, of course, a nearly life-long drug addict.

During his life, De Quincey was known for many works, but *Confessions* remains his most enduring. With its focus on subjective experience and individualism, its obsession with dreams and archetypes, and its oscillation between emotional extremes, it's a narrative that sits confidently beside the works of other English-language Romantic movement authors like Mary Shelley, Emily Brontë, and Walter Scott—as well as those by fellow opium users John Keats and Samuel Taylor Coleridge. (De Quincey was an acolyte of glorious poet and miserable addict Coleridge, who tried to warn him away from the clutches of the joy plant.)

Confessions came out some years after De Quincey moved from being a long-term recreational user of opium to a confirmed addict. The book—which, among other things, ponders withdrawal and addiction, and opium's effect on memory and imagination—was translated into French and adapted by Baudelaire, making it a literary inspiration for the Francophone Romantic world as well. *Confessions* and his other works have influenced generations of writers. An essay demonstrating De Quincey's style of black humour, "On Murder Considered as One of the Fine Arts," inspired Edgar Allan Poe as he essentially invented the detective novel. (Poe's work in turn inspired Sir Arthur Conan Doyle's creation of Sherlock Holmes, bringing us full circle.) Jorge Luis Borges considered De Quincey an influence, and Hector Berlioz's *Symphonie fantastique* was based on *Confessions*.

De Quincey first took opium for relief from a blindingly painful toothache—or possibly trigeminal neuralgia—on the advice of a college acquaintance. It was a wet Sunday in London, and he had been in agony for nearly three weeks. On Oxford Street he saw the shop of a druggist—that "unconscious minister of celestial pleasures"—and went in to purchase his first, fateful dose. He returned to his lodgings and downed it:

> That my pains had vanished was now a trifle in my eyes: this negative effect was swallowed up in the immensity of those positive effects which had opened before me—in the abyss of divine enjoyment thus suddenly revealed. Here was a panacea, a *pharmakon nepenthes* for all human woes; here was the secret of happiness, about which philosophers had disputed for so many ages, at once discovered: happiness might now be bought for a penny, and carried in the waistcoat pocket; portable ecstacies might be

had corked up in a pint bottle, and peace of mind could be sent down in gallons by the mail-coach.

This was the beginning of a love affair that lasted half a century.

From his very first, revelatory experience until his death nearly sixty years later, the Opium Eater drank his opium, as laudanum: a tincture of opium in alcohol commonly sold as an over-the-counter medicine. Although he made his name through publication of the scandalous *Confessions*, De Quincey was not doing anything even remotely scandalous when he first tried the stuff. Opiate medication was widely available—then, as now, at the drugstore, among other places—and it was relatively cheap. This made pain relief, measured in mere grains of opium or drops of opium in tincture, accessible to the working poor who could not afford wine or spirits, as De Quincey noted of a trip he took back to Manchester:

> I was informed by several cotton manufacturers, that their work-people were rapidly getting into the practice of opium-eating; so much so, that on a Saturday afternoon the counters of the druggists were strewed with pills of one, two,

or three grains, in preparation for the known demand of the evening.

I TOO REMEMBER when I started taking opioids. As I write this, it's been over four years. I expect I felt more self-conscious getting my first dose than De Quincey did, since tramadol requires not only a non-renewable prescription but the display of valid photo ID to the pharmacist.

If you have ever had a toothache like De Quincey, or dental surgery, you understand how quickly one can become desperate for relief. Having some sort of time limit on suffering makes it endurable. It's the same way that running a marathon is tolerable because you know that it will eventually end. Every step gets you closer to relief.

I don't think I'm a lightweight. I like to believe that I'm an expert on pain, thanks to hours devoted to close study of it during the births of my two children—one at home, one in hospital, neither with painkillers. Those experiences taught me that the most intense pain imaginable can be tolerated for a time, and that the way we experience that pain—empowering, terrifying, humbling—can vary dramatically.

And so even childbirth, the most painful thing commonly experienced, doesn't work as an objective measure. There are other sorts of pain, harder to describe. Chronic or recurring pains are insidious. They eat away at energy, optimism, endurance, sense of self. More relevant than a measurement or even a description of pain, then, is the completely subjective impact it has on one's thoughts, behaviour, and physical health. Pain above a "level 5"—moderate pain that dominates your thoughts and to which you cannot adapt, according to one scale designed to measure it—frequently results in temporary personality disorders. At higher levels that continue without relief, personality disorders are almost ubiquitous and suicide is common.

♩

IT IS PAIN that now regularly pushes me back to depression—a long-time acquaintance I was happy to forget when pregnancy and breastfeeding turned out to be miracle cures for my apparently hormonal woes. It is as bad as I'd remembered it. If pain were a substance it would be a dangerous, mind-altering one indeed.

But a quest for pain relief that settles on opioids

can bring an escape that is more than just physical, as Thomas De Quincey (and I) discovered. As the first person to write publicly and in detail in English about the inner experience of taking opium, De Quincey was to become the archetypal drug-dependent, tormented-but-inspired artist, and the progenitor of a whole new genre of literature—the addiction confessional—later taken up by literary junkies like William Burroughs, Irvine Welsh, Jim Carroll, and many others. And yet, his description is precise and unique-sounding rather than stereotypic. It's also utterly resonant with my experience of tramadol:

> The town of L—represented the earth, with its sorrows and its graves left behind, yet not out of sight, nor wholly forgotten. The ocean, in everlasting but gentle agitation, and brooded over by a dove-like calm, might not unfitly typify the mind and the mood which then swayed it. For it seemed to me as if then first I stood at a distance, and aloof from the uproar of life; as if the tumult, the fever, and the strife, were suspended; a respite granted from the secret burthens of the heart; a sabbath of repose; a resting from human labours. Here

were the hopes which blossom in the paths of life, reconciled with the peace which is in the grave; motions of the intellect as unwearied as the heavens, yet for all anxieties a halcyon calm: a tranquility that seemed no product of inertia, but as if resulting from mighty and equal antagonisms; infinite activities, infinite repose.

Please compare that with the following description of tramadol given by drug user "J.C." on an online forum:

> It's as if the most comfortable, softest, pink blanket is being wrapped around me in both a physical and emotional way. It is like laying back and talking with my best friend. It's like walking outside on the first day of summer and smelling the fresh cut grass. My problems have not disappeared, I have not escaped them, but the little annoyances of life have had the volume turned down a notch. Tramadol has often giving me the opportunity to reflect and feel optimistic about the future [...]
>
> The great thing about tramadol, however, is that it does not inhibit my activities at all. It

doesn't make me want to just lie on the couch like marijuana, or immediately run around the world like amphetamines. It just feels natural to continue to do, whatever it is that I do. Doing work is fine, conversations are great, sports are fun, there are hardly any activities that I can think of that Tramadol detracts from.

At twenty, Thomas De Quincey left his desultory studies at Oxford every three weeks or so to travel to London, where he would indulge in laudanum, theatre, opera, and long, rambling walks through the ancient city streets. The opiate was an essential enhancer, instilling a peaceful curiosity amid the urban tumult.

As it happens, I was also in London at about the same time in my life. Just before my twentieth birthday, I worked for six weeks in a laboratory at St. Mary's Hospital. (Also, coincidentally, this is where heroin was first synthesized, back in 1874.) Like De Quincey, but more sober and more cautious, I wandered through the city. I was in the first throes of what was eventually diagnosed as major depression. I was treated with antidepressants the following year. And yet my state of mind at that point was probably like that of young Thomas: open to everything, romantic, melodramatic, unstable, desperate to take it all in. I like to imagine how it was for him then. The dark buildings and gilding late-afternoon light, the vast and noisy variety of people of all appearances and conditions, the cobbled streets that wind like hilly labyrinths up and down and around. The grandeur of intricate stonework everywhere. Rotting timbers, memories of plague.

Just my height—a bit *under* five feet—and slight, De Quincey was sensitive and precocious, with a blazing talent at languages. He was often torn, like me, between a desire to please and conform and an equally strong attraction to rebellion and iconoclasm. "I used often," he writes, "on Saturday nights, after I had taken opium, to wander forth, without much regarding the direction or the distance, to all the markets and other parts of London to which the poor resort of a Saturday night, for laying out their wages."

On these "long, rambling nights amongst London's working class, De Quincey enjoyed the drugged bliss of both sympathy and separation," writes his biographer, Robert Morrison. "In knitting together drugs, intellectualism, unconventionality, and the city, he maps in the countercultural figure of the bohemian. Decades before Edgar Allan Poe and

Charles Baudelaire, he emerges as the first *flâneur*, high and anonymous, graceful and detached, strolling through crowded urban sprawls trying to decipher the spectacles, faces, and memories that reside there."

De Quincey describes two types of laudanum high. Immersion in an interesting crowd, or attendance at the opera, for example, are made just that much more exquisite under the influence of laudanum. But there is a second level of high where, he says, it is good to be alone in order to fully luxuriate in the sensation. Although the Opium Eater seems to have been the first person to write about deliberately selecting experiences that will be enhanced by opiates, or that will themselves enhance the opiate high, or that somehow together will create an aesthetic and emotional synergy, he's certainly not been the last. And by this I don't just mean avant-garde literati. On online forums, drug users—including prescription users who are genuinely suffering from pain and taking opioids at normal, prescribed doses—repeatedly describe particular music or social settings that seem to enhance the overall experience.

I have now mixed morphine and live theatre, morphine with intellectual café chats, morphine with art; hydromorphone with intense one-on-one friend conversation and (on a different occasion) with salsa dancing; and tramadol with an El Greco exhibit, a ballet about Vaslav Nijinsky's descent into madness, and watching Brazil beat Panama at soccer. It has also made rolling out coils of clay in a ceramics class particularly hypnotic.

DOROTHY WAS LULLED to sleep in her field of poppies in Oz and lucky to wake up. The brilliant red of the opium poppy, *Papaver somniferum*, has long been linked to death-like sleep or sleep-like death. Fields of poppies covering hundreds of thousands of acres supply the raw material for millions of opioid prescriptions and provide that ambiguous, tenuous exit from the struggles of life. Usually it's a temporary reprieve. Too often it's permanent.

Celebrities die of illegal opioids in droves. The less well known may also die with needles in their arms, or with bottles of prescribed liquid morphine in their medicine cabinets. Barbara Hodgson's book *In the Arms of Morpheus* looked at the early history of morphine and opium use in medical preparations in Europe and North America. "Fortunately today, since other, non-addictive drugs are available, morphine is limited to short-term use and to palliative care, and dependence on it through medical application is rare," she wrote. Hodgson's book was published in 2001, but this statement was not entirely true then, and it's certainly not true a decade and a half later.

Since the early 1990s, pharmaceutical companies have engaged in heavy marketing of opioid painkillers, developing and promoting dozens of new varieties. As a result, prescriptions for them have surged. Drugs once restricted to mostly in-hospital, intravenous, short-term, and palliative or post-operative use are now prescribed in lower (but often escalating) doses over the very long term to patients living with enduring pain. Unsurprisingly, unintentional deaths due to prescription opioid overdoses have also quadrupled in the U.S. over this period. The development has been gradual but accelerating and has flown largely under the popular radar for around twenty-five years. It's a situation that in some ways mirrors the widespread and haphazard use of opiate-based medicine in the nineteenth century.

Study after study points to galloping use of opioids—particularly in North America and Australia—to treat a wide range of afflictions. This surge is often reported in the news inaccurately, incompletely, and with breathless alarm. It's "a problem." It's "a rash." It's "a flood." It's "an epidemic." The "painkillers are killing us."

But the headlines are hyperbole mixed with truth. What is true is that more people are now becoming addicted to prescribed opioids, whether their own or someone else's; more people are seeking treatment for physical dependency (different from addiction) as well as actual addiction; and more people are dying of overdoses of prescription opioids.

Some fifteen million people worldwide are dependent on opiates. An increasing number of these use prescription opioids. (Not all opioids are included in the published data. Tramadol, for example, is not among the six major prescription opioids whose use is tracked by the International Narcotics Control Board—so actual numbers are considerably higher.) The World Health Organization estimates that around 69,000 people die of opioid overdoses each year.

The estimate includes illegal drugs like heroin as well as accidental overdoses of prescribed drugs—and accidental overdoses of drugs—hydromorphone, say—that are legally prescribed to *some*one, but taken by someone else. It is also made blurry by including drugs like fentanyl that are legally prescribed but are also illicitly produced and sold for recreational use, and may be used unwittingly (by someone who thinks they're taking illegal cocaine, or oxycodone that is legal but often procured for illicit use).

It's hard to keep track because the ultimate cause of death is not always obvious, either. But given the numbers of users and widespread availability of opioids, the grim global overdose statistics are not surprising. In North America alone it is estimated that around 2.1 million Americans—and some 200,000 Canadians—are currently addicted to legal opioid painkillers—these two countries being far and away their greatest consumers.

I have been on tramadol for nearly five months. I was working for four hours a day, I am now doing 10–12 hour days, I concentrate all day long and work performance is effective. My identity has been unchained from desperation and loss of soul. I can once again feel deep emotions, happiness, contentment, enjoyment from achieving good result with my work—on tramadol, it is not the sick kind of happiness as on amphetamines. It is natural—I also get down when there is a

reason. Most of the days, although, I feel extreme happiness for having come through [...] I am in balance, I am free, I am positive and most of all, I am myself—a whole identity.

— A post by a drug-use forum member

IN NEW YORK I make the shift to taking tramadol twice a day, every day. In the process, I have the striking insight that it is better to feel good than to feel bad. I wander with my friend Sonia—she high only on life—around Manhattan galleries and streets, discover magical cafés, have long conversations about art and life.

We are nearly forty. But we once did the same thing as privileged young wanderers fresh from our first year of university, when we backpacked in Paris together partway through my London laboratory contract. Then, red wine acted as a more conventional colourant to our Bohemian experience. I remember one long nighttime walk to our hostel home. We rambled on enthusiastically about life, about art, about art and life, and life as art. About commitment to social justice causes. About living with intensity. All as one does when one is nineteen and lucky and backpacking in Paris. Of course, we had experienced nothing. Nothing!

Now, wandering aimlessly in the West Village after the bruising experiences of adulthood, we end up after midnight on a quiet street. We notice a restaurant that looks as if it's closing. It turns out that it is open, dusky, impossibly romantic. There are just a couple of patrons finishing their dinners in the back. There is a grand piano, old portraits. The building is a carriage house built in 1767, some years before Thomas De Quincey was born across the sea. As we sit at the bar, the upwell of good feeling becomes almost overwhelming.

"Right now," I say, straining to put this into words, "I feel like there is just as much possibility and adventure in life as I felt all those years ago in Paris."

As De Quincey established, there is nothing better than wandering anonymously through a great and diverse city. The drug is not necessary. But it certainly is complementary. Getting lost, you find yourself.

DE QUINCEY CAME to prominence during the height of the English Romantic era, which stretched roughly from the late 1700s to around 1850. Robert

Morrison, his most recent major biographer, writes that "The Opium Eater is bookish, dreamy, and aloof, yet urban, street-smart, and with a keen interest in the macabre."

This sketch of De Quincey could apply to every Romantic. You can spot them by their interest in emotional extremes, in the morbid or melodramatic, and in the action of dreams and fantasies. Romanticism is marked by individualist subjectivity as well as its flip side—fascination with the exotic or Other.

The Romantic craze started, believed Scottish surgeon Thomas Trotter, with dependence on stimulants like coffee and tea—gateway substances along the slippery cobblestone path to the opium den. The new generation of "Romantics," he wrote, were afflicted by "the nervous disposition formerly the privilege of poets, artists, and aristocrats." How much worse, then, the tumultuous, sensation-seeking temperament of the *actual* Romantic-era poet or artist!

While biographers may argue about whether Keats's "Ode on Indolence"—

> *Ripe was the drowsy hour;*
> *The blissful cloud of summer-indolence*

> *Benumb'd my eyes; my pulse grew less and less;*
> *Pain had no sting, and pleasure's wreath no flower*

—arose from direct experience or not, there is no doubt that English literature in the nineteenth century was absolutely drenched in laudanum. The list of historical users includes a Who's Who of Romantic authors: Lord Byron, Percy Bysshe Shelley, Bram Stoker. Elizabeth Barrett Browning, Charlotte Brontë. It also includes later and perhaps less-expected figures like *Little Women* author Louisa May Alcott, a morphine addict, and Florence Nightingale—that nursely icon of devoted self-sacrifice—who regularly injected herself with morphine during the Crimean War. "I could not get through the day without this wonderful little pick-me-up," she once wrote.

Opium was just one factor at play. Tuberculosis was another. Like ankylosing spondylitis, infection with *Mycobacterium tuberculosis*—the classic microbe of the Romantics—often struck young people in their prime. A second-century description of pulmonary tuberculosis gives the image:

> The youth with the croaking voice...the extreme wasting, the nails crooked and brittle, the eyes deeply sunk in their hollows but

> brilliant and glittering...the lassitude coupled with foolish gaiety...the shoulder blades like the wings of the birds.

Bright eyes, dreamy indolence alternating with animated conversation, and bodies bespeaking indifference to food—these also characterize what the French refer to as the *opiomane*. By the nineteenth century, prevalent tuberculosis and prevalent use of opium together provided the basis of the archetypal Romantic. Opium, morphine, and heroin eased the tuberculotic sufferings and the passing of Frédéric Chopin, Aubrey Beardsley, Franz Kafka, Katherine Mansfield, George Orwell, and D.H. Lawrence.

John Keats was less fortunate. The great poet, whose work De Quincey later championed as a critic, died of tuberculosis like his brother and mother before him. In his last days, an unusually concerned friend hid from him the laudanum that could have eased his bloody cough and pain. He died in agony, just twenty-one.

Of course, of course, yes of course: drugs are more likely to be detrimental than improving to literature or art. And yet, some undeniably beautiful and passionate work arose from that drowsy hour—and its release from pain.

WELL BEFORE PAIN became an issue for me—always, in fact—I have dealt with setbacks by trying, not always successfully, to follow the writer Neil Gaiman's advice: "Husband runs off with a politician? Make good art. Leg crushed and then eaten by mutated boa constrictor? Make good art. IRS on your trail? Make good art. Cat exploded? Make good art." The breakup, the breakdown, the lousy boss, the crummy landlord, the diagnosis. They're all experiences that I can one day turn into writing. That desire to produce something, anything, that feels meaningful becomes more urgent as the setbacks increase.

So much literature has speculated about the uncertain relationship between opioid drugs and art. Art certainly acts, like drugs, as a form of short-term relief, and helps me put routine pain into perspective. Even better, it's comforting to find that my experience makes me (or lets me fancy myself) part of the long lineage of speculation on the relationship between art and drugs. Still, my own experiences have left me confused about whether opioid-based pain relief—or the other, infamous effects of opium-related drugs—actually improves my creative processes. And about whether pain itself makes me a better writer or a worse one. All I know is that both opioids and writing seem to have become vital to my existence.

Sometimes I imagine my ambitions as circus lions circumscribed by rings of fire. The fire is pain. Pain causes physical limitations; eats at my fragile sense of optimism; confuses my thoughts and imperils my livelihood; deadens the association-making ability from which creative work emerges. Pain makes me strained and cranky as I try to play with my two young children, who can absorb depression just as they thirstily absorb every other influence.

Endurance is possible, but endurance on its own does not equal a full, contributing life. Our purpose in life is not, cannot be, simply to suffer.

I HAVE SEVERAL times made conscious decisions about mind-altering drugs. The film *Trainspotting* came out in 1996, when I was nineteen. By the time I saw it, I was just learning that depression was an issue for me. The movie was my first introduction to heroin and I immediately understood that it was dangerous for me precisely because it seemed so attractive, attractive as other drugs I'd heard of—marijuana, cocaine, LSD, alcohol—had never been.

So—not that they were handing out syringes on the way out of the movie theatre, but just in case—I resolved at that moment never to try it, or anything like it. A decade and a half later, my inadvertent and unsought experience of drugs has confirmed my instinct that opioids are "my" drug. I echo De Quincey's vehemence in distinguishing between the calm glow of opium and true intoxication:

> First, then, it is not so much affirmed as taken for granted, by all who ever mention opium, formally or incidentally, that it does or can produce intoxication. Now, reader, assure yourself, *meo periculo*, that no quantity of opium ever did or could intoxicate. As to the tincture of opium (commonly called laudanum), *that* might certainly intoxicate if a man could bear to take enough if it; but why? Because it contains so much proof spirit, and not because it contains so much opium.

Certainly, opioids, unless you take enough to make you drowsy, do not distort thinking. They relieve pain and elevate your mood. This is equally true of Tylenol 3 with codeine, of fentanyl, and of heroin. Though they may be sedative—and numerous users, including me, also note paradoxical stimulant effects—they are not depressants like alcohol. No slurry words or fumbled movements. No coke-like jerkiness.

Patients taking doses prescribed for chronic pain would normally be perfectly composed and lucid, entirely normal. A little sleepy, maybe, or conversely, a little animated. The late, great Oliver Sacks describes in *Hallucinations* his experience—as a thirty-second birthday gift to himself—of injecting a significant quantity of morphine pilfered from his physician parents' medical supplies:

> Within a minute or so, my attention was drawn to a sort of commotion on the sleeve of my dressing gown, which hung on the door. I gazed intently at this, and as I did so, it resolved itself into a miniature but microscopically detailed battle scene. I could see silken tents of different colors, the largest of which was flying a royal pennant [...] I lost all sense of this being a spot on the sleeve of my dressing gown, of the fact that I was lying in bed, that I was in London, that it was 1964.

> Before shooting up the morphine, I had been reading Froissart's *Chronicles* and *Henry V*, and now these became conflated in my hallucination. I realized that what I was gazing at from my aerial viewpoint was Agincourt, late in 1415, that I was looking down on the serried armies of England and France drawn up to do battle. And in the great pennanted tent, I knew, was Henry V himself [...]
>
> I glanced at my watch. I had injected the morphine at nine-thirty, and now it was ten. But I had a sense of something odd—it had been dusk when I took the morphine; it should be darker still. But it was not. It was getting lighter, not darker, outside. It *was* ten o'clock, I realized, but ten in the morning. I had been gazing, motionless, at my Agincourt for more than twelve hours.

While a magical experience, Sacks resolved not to repeat it. One could easily dream one's life away. The few times I have tried my own modest, oral dose of morphine have not gone very well. At a very low dose, it does nothing. At double that dose, still low, it relieves pain; instills a heaviness that feels almost muscular, and paradoxically painful, even; induces great lassitude; makes time pass mysteriously. I'm drowsy, but when I try to rest my sleep is fragmented and haunted by distressing scraps of dreams.

I think Sacks is right: morphine, though helpful for dying, does not seem conducive to actually living.

MY FRIEND EMILY and I lie in the grass in the park on a chilly, sunny fall day. I pick at bits of grass as I try to explain my frustration at endless pain, at the limits it puts on my capacities, on the scope of my life.

"When the alarm goes off in the morning," I tell her, "my first feeling is of dread. I'm thinking about the amount of work I'm going to put into just sitting up. You'd rather not wake up."

Em suggests antidepressants, not for the first time. I explain that tramadol feels very antidepressant when I take it. (In fact, it has been investigated for use as a legitimate antidepressant.) Yes, I am depressed, but for the first time—notwithstanding many years, now long behind me, of not-very-effective medications—I can decide when to make that leaden hopelessness go away.

Extracts of opium, and its synthesized imitations, bind to our mu-opioid receptors—proteins present in the brain, spinal cord, intestinal tract, and elsewhere in the body. It took until 1974 for scientists to discover that we produce our very own opioids, called endorphins. The word was a neologism, a short form of "endogenous morphine," because we knew about morphine before we knew that we—clever creatures that we are—produce these magical molecules ourselves, in the brain and pituitary gland. Indeed, the receptors for opioids and endorphins have been part of our genetic makeup since our ancestors first developed backbones 450 million years ago.

So exercise is a natural form of pain relief and mild euphoria. A half an hour of running is, for me, as for many others, a reliable way to emerge from the enervating fog of depression. I'm lucky in the nature of my spine disease, at least in that regard: one of AS's diagnostic features is that stiffness and pain worsen with rest and improve with exercise. Stretching, strengthening and cardiovascular exercise are fundamental to treatment and improved outcomes.

While I can't stand for more than five minutes or sit for more than ten without pain and obvious discomfort, I can run for quite a long time on a soft indoor track. Psychologically speaking, this is life-saving. (On real morphine I'm far too lazy for exercise—but I have learned that tramadol mixed with endogenous morphine from a long run is a glorious combination.) I'd heard of people becoming addicted to exercise and had understood it as a mild mania for being fit. In fact, there is a recognized disorder called "exercise addiction" and at least some evidence suggests that the pain relief and euphoria produced by exertion can create a pleasure-seeking feedback loop. In some people this is associated with body dysmorphia, eating disorders, and control issues, but in most this is a mild and beneficial dependency—rather than the sort of thing that leads to robbing sneaker stores at gunpoint.

Will Self, the tall and cadaverous British novelist and essayist, is a former heroin addict. He was once hired by the U.K.'s *Observer* newspaper on the strength of his reputation as an exceedingly literate junkie (and later fired after he quietly snorted heroin in the bathroom of Prime Minister John Major's campaign jet). Self is also a walker, covering heroic distances measured in the tens of kilometres at a time. He wrote this passage many years after leaving off the smack:

> The surrealist poet Louis Aragon wrote a famous book called *Le Paysan de Paris*; in it he

describes how at unexpected moments during such a promenade, the walker, if sufficiently alive to the nuances of place and atmosphere, can experience the "moment." What exactly this "moment" is can seem a little obscure, but in essence it's the ambulatory equivalent of the sort of insights the surrealists believed they received from dreams, séances, automatic writing and other methods they used to short-circuit the deadening influence of rationality.

Self doesn't allude here to the resonance with the mental state of the opiated *flâneur*. But it is there. Walk long enough and natural opioids mingle with a pleasant sense of being lost—an ideally receptive, relaxed, and dynamic creative state. The writer Malcolm Cowley was once asked in a *Paris Review* interview if he had any tricks to get him going on his day's writing. He replied: "A lot of people use walking. I wonder if the decline of walking will lead to a decline of the creative process."

IN THE EVENING, my children are asleep and the house is hushed, save for the wonder of their little bellows-like breathing that fills our apartment. I stand by the fridge and pour myself a mug of milk. Earlier in the day, anticipating this moment, I tried to focus on the exact nature and quality of the pain I experience—wanting to go beyond aversion, to get something out of the experience, knowing that I have the power to banish it later on, when I am ready. That moment is finally here. I swallow a tramadol pill and a few pieces of dark, bitter chocolate to keep me awake for the most magical part of my day. As the pain melts away after an hour, I settle in at my desk.

Alethea Hayter, a British academic, tried to methodically tease apart the creativity innate in an artist and the creativity induced by their use of opiates. When Hayter published *Opium and the Romantic Imagination* in 1968, you could still get a prescription for heroin in the U.K.—but the dangers of heroin (long prohibited in the United States) and morphine addiction were becoming increasingly clear. She was curious about opioids' reputation for causing waking dreams, reveries, and vivid fantasies, and her book is a thorough analysis of the works of literary users of opium.

In reviewing the work of De Quincey, Keats, Poe, Collins, Coleridge, and others, Hayter concluded that opioids loosen the restrictions on creative thinking—and seem to enhance one's ability to find patterns. My own experience bears this out. Opioids seem to make it easier to derive symbols and metaphors from one's imaginings or from the raw material presented by reality. On tramadol, I range freely in my thoughts. I can draw analogies, coming up with unexpected parallels between disparate things or ideas. This effect on analogical thinking is mentioned over and over in the literature on opium.

But the precise nature of what opiates contribute to the creative process slips hazily through Hayter's fingers, beyond the conclusion that they stimulate metaphorical thinking, providing writers both with dream imagery and the means to creatively interpret it.

More important, to my mind, is the calm, playful focus I can achieve with tramadol. It's a state conducive to the odd combination of discipline and freedom that any art-making requires. That dispassionate absorption, more than the discrete thinking patterns that Alethea Hayter tried to tease out of her reading, seems to me to be the key to opioids' influence on creativity.

Of course, De Quincey himself made an important cautionary point about turning to substances for creativity. "If a man 'whose talk is of oxen' should become an opium-eater," he wrote, "the probability is that (if he is not too dull to dream at all) he will dream about oxen."

ANOTHER WHITE NIGHT—no sleep, no oxen—followed by fitful rest. Once the confusion of the morning passes, my dominant feeling is that of dread. I spend twenty minutes (the time I usually stretch while still lying down, reminding arthritic joints how to move) simply willing myself to face the day. Through the day I have the distinct sense of my face as an unsmiling mask, and I feel, both physically and metaphorically, that my skin is too thin.

In the afternoon I give in and take tramadol. After an hour that blessed warm feeling melts the stiffness, dissolving pain along with my black mood. I pick up my children from school and am able to play with them like a good mother. After reading them bedtime stories and kissing them goodnight, I lie down on the floor in the living room to meditate for ten timed minutes.

My mind quickly drifts. Visual imagery assembles itself before me. In precise detail against the clear and familiar background of my living room ceiling I can see the body of some creature, curled up and opened as for a dissection, the viscera in muted, contrasting colours. I then imagine—I am awake, not dreaming, in a sort of waking dream—another creature, smaller, crawling inside the body cavity of the first creature, curling up around the stomach or beside the liver, tucking itself in for comfort and for warmth.

I abort the meditation session before the ten-minute timer rings. This is my first taste of the notoriously dark opioid-induced reverie.

Thomas De Quincey's reveries—something between dreams and hallucinations—were the result of withdrawal at times, and, at others, of using laudanum. They were fearsome, but their imaginative power is remarkable. In his dreams, he writes in the *Confessions*,

> I was buried for a thousand years, in stone coffins, with mummies and sphynxes, in narrow chambers at the heart of eternal pyramids. I was kissed, with cancerous kisses, by crocodiles; and laid, confounded with all unutterable slimy things, amongst reeds and Nilotic mud.

A frightened obsession with crocodiles—representing perhaps a xenophobic Orientalism, or contrasted with the loving innocence of children, or simply a representation of all that is horror—became a recurring theme in his reveries, in his withdrawal nightmares, and in his writing:

> The cursed crocodile became to me the object of more horror than almost all the rest... All the feet of the tables, sofas, &c., soon became instinct with life: the abominable head of the crocodile, and his leering eyes, looked out at me, multiplied into a thousand repetitions; and I stood loathing and fascinated.

The terrifying image of a coach driver transformed in his imagination into such a beast—a venerable croc, in a livery of scarlet and gold—haunts De Quincey's other great work, *The English Mail-Coach*.

As for me, I have occasionally experienced other waking dreams. Once during a yoga class I imagined riding a flying carpet. The Persian rug pattern, the way it billowed toward me from the air below, a cool feeling from the wind and most of all a frightened exhilaration: it was far more real and surprising than an imagined scene, but more within my conscious control than a dream. That one was a gift.

OVER THE PAST eight years I have regularly been asked to rate various aspects of my pain—along with fatigue and resulting psychological distress—according to those one-to-ten scales mentioned earlier. (On one such scale—there are many—ten represents unbearable, unimaginable suffering, the sort that would quickly cause one to black out; one represents no pain: "feeling perfectly normal.") It's a frustrating exercise. Both mental and physical pain are difficult to quantify.

They are best expressed in metaphors: the dark hole, the cliff, the vise, the hot poker, the black dogs. Or in ambiguous phrases evoking the senses: heavy, fine and needle-like, wide or very bright. Loud and metallic. Electric. Soft and creeping. Or more like concrete, like lead, like spiders.

Pain studies could be like wine connoisseurship: "It started with a bouquet of creeping unease, then a full, bloody, vigorous sensation followed by a lingering ache."

So I write this, again, under the influence.

It's a release that I've earned through the sheer effort of waiting for it all day. At last I take the pill, and I begin to focus intently on the pain in my neck and down my back—waiting for the magic moment when it begins to melt away. I watch, feel, and wait. Minutes pass. Is it gone? I think I feel it leave. But no. The pain is still there.

Then, as it always does, at almost exactly the one-hour mark, something shifts. The ropey muscles of the neck that pull my head forward, the tight muscles around my hips, mid-back, and sacroiliac joints (in an X-ray you can see the erosion)—they all seem to loosen at last. I sigh audibly, letting my shoulders fall. I stand up straighter. Gravity stops pounding me into submission. All at once, I seem able to inhale more oxygen than usual. That breath is rich and deep. I'm also breathing more slowly than usual.

I close my eyes almost unconsciously. When I let them close, just for a moment, there's a pleasant weight on my eyelids, as if I were falling into a dreamless, restorative sleep. At the same time I seem to float, perhaps on a pool raft drifting on saltwater waves, with a sort of inner buoyancy. It is wonderful.

I could stay in it forever, like those Victorian gentlemen found after days by worried families—prostrate upon a back-alley opium den couch, obscured in a cloud of stale smoke.

But I open my eyes after a moment because in the infinite peace and wisdom now upon me—right now—I also see my goal: to write, to create, clearly and without stress.

First physical pain recedes, and then emotional pain. I was depressed, and now I am not.

Nothing is hazy or distorted or vague. There is no drunkenness, no lack of balance or blurring. I can once again see all the little worries and big angsts in my life from a bearable distance. And now, taken a little out of myself, I can also see and feel compassion for other people's struggles, am interested once again in their stories. For these few hours I have regained the essential human characteristic of someone who is well and flourishing: a healthy curiosity about everything that is not me.

Not least, the thread of thought I want to track down and record in writing plays out smoothly and I can follow it. Peaceful, concentrated work is the best opioid side effect of all.

I close my eyes again. There are endless variations in the texture of good feelings that keep me here, happily working at my desk. Every time I close my eyes—every time I inhale, deeply, then exhale—these feelings are intensified. This eye-closing, this looking within: it's a subtle action which, over a group dinner or in a café, I've sometimes caught friends catching, to my shame.

But then, why should I feel ashamed?

I've since learned, on online forums where drug users and abusers share their experiences, that this is called "nodding" or "nodding out." The term is also used simply to describe sleeping or the sleepiness associated with the drug—and more generally "being on the nod" is long-used slang for a calm and dreamy opioid high. "Nod" is the Hebrew root of the word for "to wander." The term may refer to the involuntary dropping of the chin into a literal nod, but it carries, too, associations with the Biblical land of Nod and all manner of remixed cultural notions: wandering, desires, creativity, sleep, dreams.

SUNNY MORNING, BUSY street in Toronto's Little Italy. Alam, the server at the Gatto Nero restaurant nods hello and brings me my coffee, black. Notebook open on the glass-topped, black cat–inscribed table,

I sit cross-legged and shift position every few seconds. Rattle rattle in my backpack: a pen and that little bottle of pills. In my jacket pocket I sometimes feel for its slim plastic cylinder and child-proof top as if I were Gollum fingering for my precious. I order a croissant and begin to work—the expectation of pain relief enough to get me happily through the next hour. In the same vein, the always-ailing Marcel Proust began his day with coffee, a croissant, and some opium.

Opium. *Plus ça change, plus c'est la même chose*...only the statistics are more impressive than in Proust's time. The estimated amount of opiate raw materials needed for *legal* (that is, medical) purposes around the world for 2015 was equivalent to some 620 tonnes of morphine. Globally, including non-legal uses, we collectively consumed 6.27 milligrams of morphine per person in 2013, or over 42,000 tonnes.

That's the weight of 250 houses, 350 blue whales—or a quadrillion and a half poppy seeds.

Once you leave aside (deep breath please): the social costs of addiction; the risk of fatal overdose when drugs are taken in unsafe settings, unsafe amounts, unsafe combinations, or unsafe ways; the horrifying violence that has accompanied a profitable trade in illegal drugs; and the danger of diseases transmitted by sharing needles...set aside all that and the long-term health risks of opioids are actually slight compared to many, or even most, other medicines.

The social context of prohibition makes drugs like heroin incredibly dangerous. But it's true: at low doses, *relatively* few other long-term effects have been shown, particularly for opioids taken by mouth, even though opium has been used medicinally for thousands of years, morphine for hundreds, and even a synthetic drug like tramadol for forty years now:

> [L]egal drugs like tobacco and alcohol are directly associated with a variety of serious physical health issues, while opioids—including heroin—are not in and of themselves harmful to the body (unless too high a dose is taken).

Ah, the dose. There's the rub. The Swiss-German physician-alchemist Paracelsus—who incidentally first created tincture of opium and came up with the name *laudanum*, meaning "praiseworthy"—said it first and said it best: *Dosis facit venenum.* "The dose makes the poison."

The problem with prescription opioids is a problem of dose, in that the initial therapeutic dose rarely remains therapeutic.

Knowing this—and enjoying the mental effects while depending on the pain-relieving ones—I try, as I've said, to take tramadol sparingly. But effective pain relief requires actually using it. And so I am, like De Quincey, like Coleridge, like so many others before me, falling into the same trap of raising the effective dose.

And now I find that when I'm not feeling very, very good, I'm feeling very, very horrid.

On several occasions I have looked up the number for a local distress hotline. I dial. I hang up. Nothing to say. I'm so locked up in misery I can barely talk.

Feeling that it is somehow dangerous not to stay in touch with people on the other side of the crazy line, I text jokes to my friends. The stupider and more pointless, the better. Sometimes the absurdity actually makes me laugh. I distract myself for hours looking up jokes on the Internet. Even old chestnuts can do the trick.

> *Q. How many psychotherapists does it take to change a light bulb?*

A. Just one, but it has to really want to change.

But you can't live on stupid Internet joke forums all the time. So I take tramadol more frequently, without the drug-free days that I had previously carefully interspersed between my hours of relief.

After a few weeks or a month at a particular regular daily dosing of tramadol, the euphoria I've mentioned takes longer to set in and then becomes barely noticeable—more wishful thinking than actual relief.

In fact, after someone notes that I seem to be in pain, I note that why yes, so I am. Not only is the opioid no longer doing what it's *not* supposed to do, it's also not even offering the intermittent pain relief for which it was prescribed. I feel miserable and very bleak and I realize that I have reached a fork in the road. In order to get the effects—both pain relief and high—I need to either take less tramadol, or take more.

It took Thomas De Quincey eight years to reach the same fork. Of that time, he wrote:

> True it is that for nearly ten years I did occasionally take opium for the sake of the exquisite pleasure it gave me; but so long as I took it with this view I was effectually protected from

all material bad consequences by the necessity of interposing long intervals between the several acts of indulgence, in order to renew the pleasurable sensations.

Exquisite pleasure aside, too much pain endangers my ability to properly stretch and mobilize each precious joint. It makes it harder to exercise, harder to get out of bed and face the day. As we've come to understand that maintaining mobility and circulation are crucially important in many ailments, pain management has become key to better medical outcomes. Today, poorly controlled pain is generally considered poor medicine—as well as a failure of compassion. (The latter is a fairly modern concern, quality of life not having been a major goal of medicine in ages past. Dr. Thomas Dormandy, a pathologist and the author of *Opium: Reality's Dark Dream*, writes that "Quality of life was an invention of the Romantic Age propped up by opium.")

I don't tell my family doctor that my painkillers make me high—or alter my experience of reality—and he has never asked. In an enlightened age of medical marijuana, it wouldn't really be an appropriate question. Besides, most people taking opioids as prescribed to relieve constant pain would quickly develop tolerance and lose any euphoric sensations, making them only early, emergent properties—and as beside the point as the spontaneous orgasms one patient experienced on Parkinson's meds.

And my doctor is no fool. He prescribes small doses, limited quantities, and no automatic repeats on any prescription. I ask how to prevent developing tolerance, and he reminds me that it is better to treat pain before it gets out of control. If, or when, I become tolerant, they can rotate me to another opioid. This is a wiser solution where possible than steadily increasing the dose.

He suggests two trial options, and I choose hydromorphone, a strong opioid marketed as Dilaudid. He writes me a prescription for just ten half-doses. People react quite differently to different opioids: one may produce nausea, another constipation, another itching. It's therefore sensible to let a patient try more than one in a controlled way. I actually just want to know that tramadol will go back to feeling the way it felt before, but I can't figure out how to discreetly ask the question.

Dilaudid is seven-and-a-half times stronger, milligram for milligram, than morphine. It has been implicated in many overdose deaths. I start on a miniscule dose. Typically (or ideally) a doctor will begin a patient on the minimum dose of an opioid and gradually increase it until it brings adequate pain relief. Hydromorphone is considered extremely addictive, and the opioid that (according to those in a position to know) most closely approximates the experience of heroin. The intense good feelings it's giving me this very moment as I write this back that up. I began to feel shivers of pleasurable sensation after about forty minutes.

But, like morphine (and unlike tramadol), it is poorly absorbed through the GI tract, which limits the intensity. Just as other patients using it for pain report in online forums, it doesn't seem to me to cause mental cloudiness. Neither, though, do I feel the opening of possibilities that I get with tramadol. Its pain-relieving effect is also very short-lived. On another occasion, Dilaudid seems to do little for the pain, and I increase the dose. I feel the soreness dissipate a little and a small burst of positive energy pushes me out of the house. I make it on time to meet friends at the Jean-Michel Basquiat exhibit at the art gallery—yes, the Basquiat who died in 1988 at twenty-seven, in New York, of a heroin overdose. But despite a slight dreaminess and some relief in my spine, I soon find it too painful to stand. While my friends view the paintings I'm reduced to crouching in a corner.

EVERY TWO YEARS or so, we visit my in-laws and large extended family in Mexico City. I usually make a pilgrimage to the sun-lit, fantastically coloured Casa Azul, the former home of Mexican painter Frida Kahlo and now a museum dedicated to her art and life. I've been fascinated by Kahlo's life story since my first trip there in 2002.

Through her life, Kahlo, who died in 1954, had numerous operations on a spine and pelvis forever damaged by a horrific trolley accident. Her life was filled with hour upon hour of excruciating, demoralizing pain. Through her treatments, she became addicted to painkillers (morphine and meperidine, an opioid marketed as Demerol) as well as alcohol, which she also used for pain relief. "I tried to drown my sorrows," she wrote, "but the damned things learned to swim."

So far as I know, Kahlo never heard of De Quincey, but her life reads as one great Romantic oscilloscope graph: soaring highs and subterranean lows. She might be considered the patron saint of artsy-people-who-suffer-back-pain-and-depression-relieved-only-by-reliance-on-drugs.

"I never lost my spirit," she wrote of a period spent

in the hospital near the end of her life, her beloved husband Diego Rivera ensconced for a time in a hospital room beside hers. "I always spent my time painting because they kept me going with Demerol, and this animated me and it made me feel happy." This period—enlivened by the rare presence of unreliable Rivera, and by prescription drugs—was one of many fleeting moments that Kahlo snatched from a life otherwise dominated by physical and mental suffering.

Seeing a painting in a gallery, or in the artist's own home or studio, is quite different from looking at it in a book or on a screen. You realize that an actual person—imagining, dreaming, suffering, working—held the brush, made each stroke, set down her brush in weary despair, looked out the window at the sculpture garden, back inside at the anatomy textbooks, the ceramic tiles, the bottle of tequila, or the hypodermic needle. In her diaries, you can see how Kahlo endlessly tried to reason with herself, to find hope when feeling low. She lived large when her health permitted it, collecting illustrious friends and lovers. She also collected votive paintings: folk paintings on tin in which people depict their real incidents of suffering. In detailed images and captions, they thank the Virgin of Guadalupe for intervening—for letting them recover after they were struck by lightning, incapacitated by polio, robbed and assaulted, or hit by a runaway horse. Or, in Kahlo's case, survived a broken spinal column, collarbone, pelvis, and foot—and had an iron handrail ram through her vagina, abdomen, and uterus.

Upon developing my own spine condition, I graduated from interest to identification with Kahlo. Like me, she took pre-med courses with the goal of becoming a doctor, but ended up (as all doctors will, sooner or later) a patient instead. She remained passionately interested in medicine, its tools, and its subject, the struggling human body, and portrayed these in gruesome detail in her paintings. She found solace and meaning in art, while being constantly frustrated by the limits imposed on her by physical and mental suffering.

In periods of great illness and pain, Kahlo dressed with extravagant care, layering on jewellery to distract herself and those around her. When feeling particularly demoralized, I copy her, wearing multiple bright necklaces. One of her paintings is a self-portrait with the spine represented as a broken column, resembling something from an ancient Greek temple. For years, I misinterpreted it for some reason to be the long barrel of a gun running up her body instead of a spine. Either way, it is a searing representation of what it feels like to have a crumbling, grumbling vertical axis where a healthy backbone ought to be.

Like De Quincey, Frida Kahlo exploited her suffering for its inherently dramatic possibilities in art. I recognize in De Quincey's lush descriptions of the pains and the pleasures of laudanum the impulse I see in myself to romanticize my experiences. In Kahlo, I recognize the desperate nature of that impulse.

SOME COMMENTATORS HAVE described Kahlo's ongoing search for medical treatment that might bring physical relief as pathological, attributing her physical symptoms to a misplaced search for love through medical intervention. This is a strain of the frequently unjustified, skeptical response that healthcare providers give to many pain sufferers, particularly women—especially women from racialized groups, or who live in poverty, or who have multiple health issues. They may be dismissed as drug-seekers, disturbed souls, or hysterical. And their pain is vastly under-treated or mismanaged, resulting in further desperation and apparently odd behaviour.

Some doctors speak of pain sufferers principally as "difficult patients" who need to be redirected, spoken firmly to, or appeased. Others talk about the "pain lobby"—a vague reference to overbearing drug marketers in cahoots with lily-livered legislators and pushover docs, along with strident patient advocacy groups. I find such voices dismissive, blindingly privileged, loose or selective with evidence, and patronizing, even as they raise valid questions about these drugs and how they are used.

For those few writers who have questioned the authenticity of Kahlo's symptoms and ongoing suffering, I can only prescribe a handrail through the vagina, if any of them have one, in hopes of provoking a more compassionate—and ultimately more clinically effective—response.

Moved by greater compassion and greater insight, Fernando Antelo, a physician, wrote:

> Frida Kahlo's life and artwork can serve as a resource for physicians who want to better comprehend the experience and dehumanizing consequences of pain. Her paintings are a medium to visualize pain and the effect of pain on the human condition. We witness the suffering, grief, and doubt in Kahlo's paintings; through them, we can contemplate the experience of pain from the perspective of the

patient. Patients living with pain are acutely aware of their bodies in ways that healthy people may not be. Pain can be discernible and persistent as well as dynamic and indefinable.

Pain, moreover, can bring about a transformation in a person that manifests both physically and mentally. Living with pain can have a paralytic effect on a person's goals and dreams, in addition to family, marriage and career. Though the practice of medicine often focuses on diagnosis, treatment and education, the role of the physician demands much more. By understanding pain as a complex phenomenon that affects many aspects of life, we as physicians can fulfill our role to comfort and heal.

Lately, when I've briefly stopped taking tramadol, I've found that I may have some physical dependence on it. After a Monday through Thursday stretch without it, I experience withdrawal symptoms: abrupt and intense depression, restless sleep, and stomach upset. I don't crave it, though, unless

I am in severe pain, so I think what I'm craving is the pain relief rather than the opioid itself. In fact, it becomes a little contest with myself to see how long I can go without. Upon giving in and taking the drug, though, it is like coming back to myself.

As addicts say, in the end I am taking the drug not for a high, but just to feel normal. Or in De Quincey's words: "Since leaving off opium, I take a great deal too much of it for my health."

I started out taking a pill for severe cramps. That turned into taking 10–20 mgs on the weekends. That turned into taking 45–60 mgs every day for the past 7 months. I am a functional addict; I work full time and have a very successful Etsy business on the side which I put hours into as a second full time job. I thought I would never be a daily user but here I am. It makes me able to work harder, and that extra money earned goes to pills. I wish I could only use on the weekends, but now there's always an excuse to use more, to be creative, to be in a good mood for my bf's birthday coming up, to go to the gym.

—Another drug-use forum post

I WRITE TO Wayne Skinner, co-author of a book called *Substance Abuse in Canada*. He's a social worker specializing in addiction at the Centre for Addiction and Mental Health in Toronto. The book reflects what is called a biopsychosocial approach to addiction. In other approaches, addiction may be viewed as a brain disease, or as a moral failing, or as a "disease" of choice, or as a life sentence meted out in one's genes. I disclose in my email that although I don't currently meet any of the definitions of addiction I'd read in his book, I do regularly take prescription opioid medication.

He replies with grave kindness, and on a cold day in January I walk the ten minutes from my house to his office in the former Provincial Lunatic Asylum. I'm quite nervous but the avuncular Skinner sets me at ease, asking about my kids and telling me about his granddaughter. We proceed to talk for two meandering, challenging hours. I explain that I am conflicted about my use of opioid medications. I also tell him that they have been a revelation in that they give me control over depression. I confide—bashfully—that while I am taking them as prescribed and in modest doses for pain, I do choose when to take them more on the basis of enjoyment, especially on quiet evenings to write.

In a way it seems that I'm insistently trying to establish myself as being "on the edge" of being an addict; gently, he pushes back, defining me with equal insistence as a person doing the best she can.

According to the biopsychosocial approach to addiction, just because something is highly pleasurable, illegal, or dangerous doesn't mean anyone who uses it will fall prey to addiction. Addiction is far more complex, and results from an individual combination of an experience feeling immediately rewarding, of biological predisposition, of availability of the pleasurable substance, of our relationships with other people, and of physical or emotional suffering that may be relieved by the behaviour or substance.

Skinner speaks generally about addiction, which includes behaviours like compulsive gambling or porn addiction. But there *are* substances—like opioids—that seem to invite dependency.

"Addictive substances are appetitive and reinforcing," Skinner says. *Appetitive*, a lovely word, in that such substances satisfy deep appetites for pleasure. And *reinforcing*, because such pleasure carves strong, memorable grooves into the psyche, particularly in people who for some reason feel they need it. "People who are opioid-dependent have higher rates of depression than in the general population. Addiction problems tend to be accompanied by mental health issues," he tells me. "For example, people with anxiety may find relief in drinking alcohol or smoking pot, while those suffering with attention deficit disorders may turn to stimulants, including cocaine, to self-medicate their symptoms."

He also mentions that conflict avoidance is an issue for many opioid users. I file that one away to worry about later.

What Skinner is saying relates to effects I observe in myself, and to what I've read about others' experiences with opioids. In my case, tramadol is appealing partly because it somehow firms up the shaky boundaries of my personality. My ego becomes vague and crushable when I'm depressed. But with tramadol it is robust, an adequate container: the expansive inner feeling it generates is soft but resilient, a protective bubble.

I think I now better understand things I've heard about serious opiate addicts—especially heroin users, who may lose interest altogether in making meaningful connections with other people. "Sometimes ah think that people become junkies just because they subconsciously crave a wee bit ay silence," wrote

Irvine Welsh of heroin addicts in *Trainspotting*. Indeed, wrapped in the gauzy cocoon of peaceful concentration that accompanies the far less intense hit of a legal, low-dose narcotic, it's not difficult to shrug off the slings and arrows of difficult people and demanding relationships—or the lack thereof.

De Quincey himself attributed his attachment to opium to childhood trauma, and spoke of it as satisfying a genuine need: "I trace the origin of my confirmed opium-eating to a necessity growing out of my early sufferings in the streets of London," he wrote.

The broader world—the one outside my head—confirms this attraction. Despite scarce published data on rates of opioid use among First Nations, Inuit, and Métis communities in Canada, a number of First Nations communities have declared community emergencies due to the prevalence of prescription drug abuse and related harms like accidental overdose and suicide, with Canada's Auditor General expressing similar concerns. Many of these communities are already suffering from relatively poor health, just one result of multigenerational trauma resulting from residential schools and a long legacy of racism, violence, and cultural genocide.

Tramadol, regarded in North America as barely

even an opioid, has become an incredibly popular street drug in occupied Palestine, as well as in other places in the Middle East. In Egypt it has surpassed cannabis and heroin as the most popular recreational drug. In Gaza, under an endless occupation where there is little or no opportunity for advancement or escape and where things lurch from crisis to crisis, people live in a constant state of tension and confinement, leavened by unique incidents of horror. No wonder that a drug that offers a deep sense of peace and elevation is appealing. In 2010, international newspapers reported that Hamas officials burned some two million of the painkiller pills in an attempt to combat rampant addiction—and, perhaps, to prevent chemically induced tolerance of the intolerable.

THE ROMANTICS HAD tuberculosis and rheumatic fever. Today, arthritis pain is one of the principal ailments driving people to use opioids. An aging population subject to osteoarthritis—as well as higher rates of chronic inflammatory diseases like rheumatoid arthritis or AS—is going to be a population with ever-higher rates of daily, maddening joint pain. According to the National Institute on Drug Abuse, "the bulk of American patients who need relief from persistent, moderate-to-severe non-cancer pain have back pain conditions (approximately 38 million) or osteoarthritis (approximately 17 million)."

But do we really *need* relief?

Pain does not have to be depressing. There are ways to distance oneself from it. The most helpful I've found is the sort of mindfulness meditation where you actually try to observe pain quite intently, noticing exactly, with curiosity, and without judgement, just what it is like. Over time, you find ways to go beyond just "I hate it, I want it to stop"—that is, to overcome aversion and attraction.

I learned this formally through a structured set of mindfulness-based stress reduction (MBSR) workshops developed by Jon Kabat-Zinn, a professor of medicine and founder of the Stress Reduction Clinic and the Center for Mindfulness in Medicine, Health Care, and Society at the University of Massachusetts Medical School. The approach is based on Buddhist principles, with the mysticism stripped out. MBSR training, sometimes combined with cognitive-behavioural psychotherapy, is now widely offered across North America for the treatment of chronic pain, anxiety, depression, and a host of other conditions.

Despite practicing mindfulness, however, I find

that it remains extremely hard to prevent ongoing pain from veering quickly into complete despair.

My New York insight is that it's better to feel good than to feel bad: I can't tell now whether this represents a passionate rebuttal to the quiet martyrdom of everyday suffering or a sign of weakness, of surrender to the most primitive drives that classify all things according to good/bad, aversion/attraction.

Opioids replace the non-judgement of mindfulness with a powerful attraction to what feels good. That attraction can lead one down a very dark hole. And yet that attractive sensation of calm observation—Rebecca Solnit's reptilian feeling—is the same empty, comfortable detachment that the experienced meditator may occasionally feel. It's equally analogous to the notion of "flow" as described by psychologist Mihály Csíkszentmihályi: the time-suspending feeling that comes from total absorption in an activity.

Flow has, like mindfulness, been popularized to death in a million positive psychology self-help books, none of which mention that opioids can get you there faster—and despite distracting obstacles like worry, sadness, or pain.

THE HOLY GRAIL for researchers and pharmaceutical companies: a non-addictive, non-dangerous opioid. They've certainly tried. The really hard part is selecting for analgesic effects while avoiding the deliciously reinforcing reward pathway. Over the decades and centuries, creators and purveyors of pharmaceuticals have enthusiastically marketed such alternatives as:

- morphine (non-addictive alternative to opium);

- long-acting oxycodone (non-addictive alternative to morphine);

- tramadol (non-addictive alternative to oxycodone);

- methadone (non-addictive alternative to heroin); and

- heroin (non-addictive alternative to morphine), among others.

More recently, rising fears about overdose and addiction rates are making former pariah drugs like marijuana seem an innocuous alternative. Indeed, cannabis is a very promising alternative or adjunct to lower doses of opioids or other drugs—but its long-term effects are largely unknown, and its effect on cognition and motor skills means that it is definitely not a good option for all pain patients. Then there is the Butrans transdermal, an opioid patch that is, in the traditionally flippant way, proposed as a less-easily abused alternative to the strong, long-acting fentanyl pain patch.

In practically every case, the marketing pressures and inducements placed on doctors and government regulators by pharmaceutical companies have been relentless and, often, shameless.

In the last few years, researchers at the Memorial Sloan-Kettering Cancer Center have announced the development of new, powerful opiate analgesics that do not cause physical dependence or reinforcing behaviour (or a number of other common opiate side effects like respiratory depression and constipation). The science behind it is interesting and based on an evolution in our understanding of the diversity of opioid receptors—but maybe only time will tell if these, or other newly developed opium-inspired painkillers, are the long-sought non-addictive opioids.

I WONDER IF I'm in some new spot on the continuum of addiction severity: the pre-addiction obsessive fascination stage. I think about my opium eating and what it all means—a lot. There is a phrase I came across when I started googling "opiate experiences" and similar terms. The phrase is "opiate naïve." It means someone who is new to using opiates (recreationally or otherwise) and has not developed any level of tolerance to the drugs. It's a good term also for my feeling upon discovering an online world of people with relatively normal lives and surprising drug habits:

> *yeah there's no way to tell how often you can use without becoming an addict. When I broke my arm I was only taking a half to maybe two percs at a time but before i knew it i was taking 20 at a time which led to shooting heroin so yeah...doesn't matter how you start out because more than likely it'll end up being an addiction. Not something you can play around with.*

As soon as *Confessions of an English Opium-Eater* was published, critics immediately voiced fears that it would inspire others to become recreational opium users and addicts. In one Sherlock Holmes story, "The Man with the Twisted Lip," Dr. Watson describes an old friend who had done just that:

> The habit grew upon him, as I understand, from some foolish freak when he was at college; for having read De Quincey's description of his dreams and sensations, he had drenched his tobacco with laudanum in an attempt to produce the same effects. He found, as so many more have done, that the practice is easier to attain than to get rid of, and for many years he continued to be a slave to the drug, an object of mingled horror and pity to his friends and relatives.

Much of what is written about opioids, including rather a lot of the medical literature, conflates the distinct terms "dependency" and "addiction." These are in turn complicated by the reality of tolerance. Those who use drugs for pain relief typically find that over time you need to take more of them to get the same analgesic effect. This is simply how opioids work. It means that you are developing tolerance, and thus require higher doses.

Physical dependence, where your body comes to depend upon the opioids and reduces its own production of endorphins, may arise more quickly than tolerance and is a separate phenomenon—although they often occur at the same time. If you stop taking the drug abruptly once you have become physically dependent on it, you then experience unpleasant withdrawal symptoms.

It's not clear what proportion of the people usually described as "addicted"—in apocalyptic-sounding news reports about the "opioid crisis"—are actually physically dependent (due to the drugs being used for treatment of long-term severe pain) without exhibiting the behavioural issues that define psychological addiction.

Still, the doctor-sanctioned escalation of doses that often occurs as patients become tolerant to their original dose represents a failure of opioids as a pain relief option. Patients end up chronically taking dangerous doses, trapped by the pains of withdrawal from exploring other options. (And opioids can occasionally, especially at high doses, actually *cause* new pain.) Prescribing opioids responsibly requires a very careful hand.

🍢

REGARDLESS OF HOW you define it, after a spate of poor health and depression incited him to start taking laudanum daily, De Quincey fell into some version of dependence, and for the rest of his life laudanum was as vital to him as food and water. He chronicled much of this less-transcendent aspect of the drug in a section of his *Confessions* entitled "The Pains of Opium."

Over and over he tried to reduce or stop completely his intake of laudanum, each time bringing on, within a few days, an atrocious list of emotional and physical withdrawal symptoms. ("Cold turkey" refers to the gooseflesh from chills that are one common symptom of opiate withdrawal; "kicking the habit" refers to restless legs, another withdrawal symptom.) Though he happily exploited his laudanum experience in his published writing, De Quincey's suffering with such symptoms of withdrawal and others—violent depression, gastrointestinal upset, terrible nightmares, insomnia, trouble concentrating, and voracious craving for the drug—was genuine and chronicled with much greater desperation in his private letters to friends.

During six months of despair induced by reduced dosages, he wrote in his private journal: "Horrible! that a man's own chamber—the place of his refuge and retreat—should betray him!...Not fear or terror, but inexpressible misery, is the last portion of the opium-eater."

Sometimes, with me as with De Quincey, it is hard to tell whether the painkiller is causing or alleviating mental distress, or whether it's not related at all. De Quincey wrote in one letter that:

> Whatever I may have been writing is suddenly wrapt, as it were, in one sheet of consuming fire—the very paper is poisoned to my eyes. I cannot endure to look at it, and I sweep it away into vast piles of unfinished letters, or inchoate essays.

De Quincey's wife Margaret and his children would sit with him as he suffered sleepless nights with the agonies of withdrawal. In his definitive biography, Robert Morrison writes,

> "Margaret attended him through these dreadful sieges of physical and spiritual despair. His sufferings frightened her, and when she witnessed the horror of his attempts to reduce his opium dosages, she was the 'first to beg me to desist.' At length De Quincey 'grew afraid to sleep'. One solution was simply to stay up the whole night and the following day. Another was to ask Margaret and the children 'to sit around me and to talk: hoping thus to derive an influence from what affected me externally into my internal world of shadows.'"

This stratagem did not work, and he battled with himself, taking increasingly high, even astonishing doses before making further agonizing but successful attempts to lower the dose—for a time. His family remained devoted, and though hectic, his family life was harmonious. (A serious and long-term addict at a time when the average man lived less than half a century, Thomas De Quincey died at the very respectable age of 74, having far outlived his long-suffering wife. He took laudanum virtually until his death.) A close reading of De Quincey's life—such as I have gleaned second-hand from the work of Robert Morrison and of Joel Faflak (curiously, both professors at universities in my home province of Ontario)—suggests that if he hadn't been continually on the verge of financial ruin due mostly to addictive *behaviours* rather than substances, his life might have been a far easier one, notwithstanding the decades-long addiction to opium.

Book buying, in fact, was the most compulsive of De Quincey's various addictive behaviours. He would spend money he couldn't afford on books, let his rooms pile up with papers, and then, overwhelmed at the task of cleaning them out, actually move out and rent new lodgings, sometimes for himself and his family, sometimes just for him to quietly live and work.

The result was that despite professional success and a steady output of published writing, he was constantly in debt, to the point that he was hounded by solicitors, legal officers, and dozens of creditors from across England and Scotland (where he lived for years). He was occasionally homeless, often in hiding, and more than once sought sanctuary for himself and his family within the six- or seven-mile circumference of Edinburgh's Holyrood sanctuary to avoid being taken into debtor's prison. Several times he was "put to the horn," in which messengers-at-arms blew three blasts on a horn in the marketplace and then denounced him by name for his debts.

A genuine eccentric,

> De Quincey often "set something on fire, the commonest incident being for someone to look up from work or book to say casually, 'Papa, your hair is on fire', of which a calm, 'Is it, my love?' and a hand rubbing out the blaze was all the notice taken". One night a maid reported with alarm that De Quincey's study was on fire. The sisters rushed downstairs, but were told by their father that they could not use water to combat the blaze, "as it would have ruined the beloved papers". Instead, De Quincey entered the room, locked the door behind him, and put the flames out with a heavy rug. "He was not a reassuring man for nervous people to live with," Florence remarked mildly. Margaret was more to the point: "for Papa, we are at a constant war with him."

WHEN THE PAIN is too grinding, I sometimes find that if I can go deeply enough into depressive words and music, no longer trying to be upbeat, I at least feel in sync. Never mind the goths. I'll take Nirvana, the Stones' "Paint it Black," a little "Toccata and Fugue in D minor."

The Romantics did not notice their suffering from a distance. They sought it out. They wallowed in it, in its texture and temperature and hue. If I go into it deep enough, maybe I can make myself like the pain.

Well, here it is. Something has seized the back of my neck and the trapezius muscles down the sides in an impossibly tight grip. It's as if someone were standing behind me, forcing me to bend. It is unbearable. I don't know what my next step will be if I stop getting regular hours of relief with tramadol. Indeed, this is becoming a demonstration not of the slippery slope or downward spiral into addiction but of the impact of ongoing severe pain on mental health.

Throwing oneself into the aesthetic feeling of misery takes a dangerous level of commitment to experience. Joel Faflak writes that aesthetes like Charles Baudelaire "read De Quincey's addiction as part of the exquisite beauty of a life lived too exquisitely, a dangerous literary existence suffused with 'an incurable melancholy.'" I'm all for *saudade*, but this is all starting to feel a little too-too exquisite to me.

I ask my rheumatologist to refer me to the Centre for Addiction and Mental Health—not for addiction treatment but because I'm feeling desperate from pain and, notably, from my despair at the limitations it puts on my activities and aspirations.

I am not managing.

As tramadol has become a less reliable, complete escape from both emotional and physical angst, I return to my range of other mental tricks. They are all mindfulness or flow strategies. I've rediscovered piano practice: despite the unpleasantness of sitting up straight, I welcome the focused distraction as my fingers move through the scales and melodies I used to know.

I draw—not to produce anything, but patiently, carefully sketching in every detail of a scene, knowing that the longer I spend on each part of the whole, the more I will be absorbed by the work and temporarily freed of awareness of pain. I exercise, forcing myself through a half an hour of unpleasant warming up of joints before a warm springiness begins to loosen up the tight and painful joints and muscles—and a mental elation (endogenous morphine!) unclouds my brain.

No matter how bad I feel, I take more and more comfort and uncomplicated joy from playing with my children—while simultaneously working hard to focus moment to moment and hide from them my tension and misery. When these strategies work, they get me through another ten minutes, another hour, another day.

Nothing so magical, so *easy*, as the opioids.

I'M ON A six-hour hike partway up a volcano, and I'm parched under the blistering sun. I'm in my early twenties, on a biology field course to Ometepe, an island in the centre of Lake Nicaragua. I forgot to bring my water bottle, have no hat, did not apply enough sunscreen and am not keeping up well with the group. But I get there, one step at a time.

What sticks in my memory, looking back, is the moment when we reached our goal, a waterfall half-way up, and our guide took oranges out of his pack and shared out the juicy segments. That simple snack tasted better than the best meal of my life. It tasted like relief, it tasted like life. I think that in the popular image of the prescription drug user, the drugs become a numbing substitute for life, but that is the opposite of my experience.

I don't know how I would manage the unrelenting, ever-surprising trek of a rich, busy family life without the sweet relief of painkillers. Sometimes I feel desperately grateful.

I CALL IN prescription refills regularly. The pharmacist—my unconscious minister of celestial pleasures—is used to my frequent visits. When the doctor once fails to renew a prescription before the long weekend, she re-sends the request, looking at my face and writing URGENT on the fax.

By overlapping doses, I finally—at the very end of the day—feel the weight of my head lift from my shoulders and the burn in my lower back ease. It is wonderful to be able to turn my head without pain or unbearable stiffness for the first time today but I have to work to keep the clear and focused dreaminess I have been claiming to feel when on tramadol.

And—testing, testing—I still feel a painful resistance if I try to lift my head back to look up in a normal way. The stiffness caused by acute inflammation in my spine is simply too much to mask anymore (or at this dose). Though I know that if I hadn't been taking tramadol I would not have been sitting down as I wrote this. Because I simply wouldn't have been able to sit down. Or, for that matter, to make dinner for my family, wash dishes, sweep crumbs off the table, or help my son floss his teeth.

In a revision to the *Confessions*—thirty years after its first publication—De Quincey sums up the ups and downs associated with both physical and psychological need for the drug, and the desire to be free of both opium and pain, as consisting of:

> [...] manoeuvres the most intricate, dances the most elaborate, receding or approaching, round my great central sun of opium. Sometimes I ran perilously close into my perihelion; sometimes I became frightened, and wheeled off into a vast cometary aphelion, where for six months "opium" was a word unknown. How nature stood all these seesawings is quite a mystery to me: I must have led a sad life in those days.

As well as being a fundamental technique for coping with pain—and depression, its mental cognate—mindfulness is one of the newer and most promising strategies for dealing with addiction and its siblings (e.g., obsessive compulsive disorder, anxiety or eating disorders). In all cases, the issue is one of unbearable sensation.

The unending stress of the Gaza occupation: sensation that comes from the external world. Childhood sexual abuse, whose trauma continues into adulthood, perhaps represents an unbearable internal sensation, and is a common element in the life histories of many serious, hard-to-treat opioid addicts. The remedy for sensations of awfulness that the human psyche—no matter how Romantic—is not well equipped to handle is detached, curious, calm, and focused observation. It's an attitude easily reached while under the influence of opioids, but one that takes hard daily practice—hourly or constant practice, even—without chemical help.

I have briefly known this feeling when writing is going really well and I lose my sense of self in the best possible way, writing down ideas that I know are sure and right, images that feel inspired, as easily as if I were merely transcribing. Not just mental stresses, but physical pain, even, become unimportant in those moments of flow, the effortlessness that comes when completely focused on creation. When I come out of this trance, two hours may have passed in what feels like seconds. Something new has been brought into the world. And I have not noticed that I was in pain.

The actor Alan Arkin writes of the craft of acting, which he describes as his addiction:

> For those few minutes I was living in a state of grace. It was a place where nothing could go wrong [...] I now lived not just for acting, for being in front of an audience, but for the possibility of that exalted experience returning. I lived for those moments when the part played me and I was completely out of the way.

As Arkin goes on to say, those moments can occur in acting, arts, sports, or other fields and must be earned by hard and persistent work—but their arrival cannot be predicted or guaranteed. Each of the artists and writers name-checked in this essay has felt it. A slang term for smoking opioids or other drugs, and the pursuit of the fleeting opioid high, is "chasing the dragon"—an evocative phrase that seems better suited to the work of art. A dragon truly worth chasing. I would do almost anything for that feeling.

I MEET MY friend Derek for lunch. I take tramadol, and it is only partway through the meal that I feel some relief from pain and can finally sit down to eat. Derek practices Shambhala Buddhism, and so it is to him that I come with the question of why my work at mindfulness isn't enough. "I spend all my energy watching my pain without judging it, and so I'm depressed that that's all I'm doing with my life," I complain, tears welling. "And then I have to watch my depression without judging *that*!"

He doesn't tell me to meditate harder. He doesn't ask me what I'm doing wrong. He gives me a careful hug. Derek is the best of Buddhists, the best of friends. "I think you need hope," he says.

Until I can prevent pain from pushing me into hopelessness, it looks like I will be relying on opioid drugs to provide daily hours of relief. At the same time, my six months on daily opioids have only helped me to prove for myself what is already known: there are no quick fixes, no matter how desperately I—or any other pain patient—may need them. A drug that works best when you take it least often is not going to be a great solution to life-long pain, unless I can find a way to mitigate the effects of enduring pain. Then I can go back to taking only occasional doses for relief—and for that wonderful, cool transcendence.

I GO THROUGH many nights with no painkillers, often waking from pain, turning over and over through the long hours in search of a comfortable position. When I wake up to the morning alarm it's with the distinct feeling that I've been hit by a truck. I'll lie in bed for a while as I contemplate turning over—then, still in bed, spend fifteen minutes stretching very, very slowly, with long pauses in between movements as I prepare myself for the next painful stretch.

I DON'T TELL my former interview subject, Wayne Skinner, that I've booked myself in at his workplace, the Centre for Addiction and Mental Health. At my intake appointment, the psychiatrist and I both gloss over the opioid question (low doses, obvious pain). I fill out yet another set of rate-your-misery questions. Hesitate over one.

"Have you ever made a plan?"

At first I don't even understand the question. Then I get it.

No, no. No! Never. Of course not.

I think about it often, but that's not a plan. I have children I love. I have many dear friends, I have family who care. I am so lucky. I have things I want to do. Far too much to live for. The intake psychiatrist turns back to his screen and types, "She endorses passive suicidal thoughts." And, "She is capable of caring for herself and is not at imminent risk of serious self-harm."

He sends me out with a list of mindfulness meditation programs to contact, recommendations that I look into mood stabilizers and antidepressants, a referral for magnetic deep brain stimulation. I wonder what I was hoping for.

I trudge homeward through Little Italy and pick up my kids.

There's old Thomas De Quincey, back in nineteenth-century London with his rooms of books and papers, his decanter of laudanum, his watchful daughters, and his hair occasionally on fire. And here, travelling across the ocean and through the years, is Mexico City. It was there, sitting in the Franciscan church in the elegant central Mexico City neighbourhood of Coyoacán, more than a decade ago, that I really fell in love with the man who would become the father of our two boys. Every old house and taco stand and cobblestone is still luminous to me with that memory. It is with that tender feeling that I return now to the Casa Azul.

Frida's house—the Blue House—is bright, highly designed, and arranged, personal. A collection of pre-Hispanic sculptures sits in the courtyard garden. Cats weave in and out. The museum is full of her paintings. As a visitor years after her death, I can hold in my mind both the pain and the magic of this art that is the pure expression of joy, often, and more often of suffering: "*Mi pintura lleva con ella el mensaje del dolor*," she said—"my painting carries with it the message of pain."

Looking at a reproduction of her illustrated diary,

you can see that near the end of her life her handwriting became lighter and looser. Her painting as well.

"The drugs she was taking," writes Christina Burrus, "in particular the Demerol, caused her to swing between euphoria and despair, also affecting the steadiness of her hand and consequently the precision of her brushstrokes. Her style, which had been a meticulous as a miniaturist's, became more relaxed as a result."

Her body, under the elaborate traditional Tehuana dresses she wore, was covered with injection scabs.

The last image in Kahlo's diary is rather like Vincent Van Gogh's final painting of crows under a menacing sky: pulsing with foreboding, devoid of hope. In her sketch, a galloping horse casts a dark shadow under a pitilessly bright day. She writes ambiguously, upon going into the hospital, "I hope the leaving will be joyful, and I hope never to return."

Frida Kahlo died of a pulmonary embolism—or, possibly, an overdose, possibly an intentional one. Indeed, pain without end—and here the distinction between physical and mental pain becomes impossible to make—may be too much to endure, even for people used to suffering. Even used to laughing at it, or with it. With the help of her dangerous and appetitive medicines, Kahlo managed to ease her pain just enough to periodically and strongly embrace life. Shortly before she died, she painted her famous, joyous still life of watermelons.

Brilliant colours, with a hand-written message: *Viva la Vida!*

To life!

Notes

page 7 "**If the entire materia medica**" Macht 1915, LXIV(6), pp. 477–481.

page 11 "**into a cool spectator or your own sensations**" Solnit 2005, p.109.

page 13 "**lying down was perhaps even more**" Sebald 2001, p.85.

page 15 "**in terms of equivalencies of morphine**" See, for example, http://emedicine.medscape.com/article/2138678-overview [accessed March 4, 2016].

page 16 "**at the Boots pharmacy in Piccadilly Circus**" Duffy 2006.

pages 16–17 "**Sherlock Holmes took his bottle**" Doyle 1986, p.107.

page 19 "**Opium! Dread agent of unimaginable pleasure and pain!**" De Quincey (Wordsworth) 1994, p.10. This Vintage Classics edition reproduces the original, tighter 1821 version rather than De Quincey's revised and lengthened later edition. All references to Thomas De Quincey where not otherwise indicated are from this edition.

pages 19–20 "**emblazon the power of opium**" De Quincey, *Confessions of an English Opium-Eater*, Wordsworth Editions, 1994, p. 10. This is a reproduction of the revised edition De Quincey published in later life.

page 20 "**the effect of the subconscious on the psyche**" As Joel Faflak discusses, among other historical themes, in his excellent introduction to Thomas De Quincey's *Confessions of an English Opium-Eater*. Broadview Editions, 2009, p.36. This reprint of the

Confessions is also based on the revised edition De Quincey issued in later life.

pages 22–23 "unconscious minister of celestial pleasures" De Quincey (ed. Faflak) 2009, p.88.

page 22 "That my pains had vanished" De Quincey (Wordsworth) 1994, p.180.

page 23 "then, as now, at the drugstore, among other places" Eli Lilly, for example—known today as the makers of Prozac—once sold tablets of camphorated tincture of opium among the huge range of completely legal, heavily marketed, and widely sold opium medicines used for a variety of common and mild ailments. Hodgson, 2001, has a fuller and beautifully illustrated account.

pages 23–24 "I was informed by several" De Quincey (ed. Faflak) 2009, p.53.

page 25 "Pain above a 'level 5'" The guidelines for the 0–10 Pain Scale, via Lucile Packard Children's Hospital Heart Center/CVICU, are explained at https://lane.stanford.edu/portals/cvicu/HCP_Neuro_Tab_4/0-10_Pain_Scale.pdf [accessed March 2, 2016].

pages 26–27 "The town of L—represented the earth" De Quincey (ed. Faflak) 2009, p.100. The town in question is Liverpool, oddly enough (Morrison 2009, p.109). Working with newly found primary sources as well as with the previously definitive biography of De Quincey by Grevel Lindop, Robert Morrison has written the most thorough account of De Quincey's life to date. My understanding of De Quincey's character and details of his life history are drawn principally from Morrison's work.

pages 27–28 "It's as if the most comfortable" Forum user J.C. writing in 2005 at https://www.erowid.org/experiences/exp.php?ID=23886 [accessed March 1, 2016].

page 29 "I used often" De Quincey 2013, p.68.

page 29 "long, rambling nights amongst London's" Morrison 2009, p.109.

pages 29–30 "In knitting together drugs" Morrison 2009, p.108.

pages 31–32 "Fortunately today, since other" Hodgson 2001, p.4.

page 32 "pharmaceutical companies have engaged in heavy marketing of opioid painkillers" None of which function in substantially different ways, however.

page 32 "unintentional deaths due to prescription opioid

overdoses have also quadrupled" See https://www.drugabuse.gov/about-nida/legislative-activities/testimony-to-congress/2016/americas-addiction-to-opioids-heroin-prescription-drug-abuse

pages 32–33 "often reported in the news inaccurately" For just a sample of the seemingly endless number of such reports, see: http://www.examiner.com/article/new-study-seeks-to-force-canada-to-face-its-opiate-problem; http://www.cbc.ca/news/canada/montreal/rash-of-fatal-overdoses-in-montreal-could-be-linked-to-fentanyl-1.2692418; http://www.denverpost.com/ci_20199285/medical-community-tries-slow-flood-painkiller-misuse; http://www.thestar.com/news/gta/2012/02/27/oxycontin_delisting_will_not_halt_ontarios_painkiller_epidemic_doctors_say.html; or http://knowmore.washingtonpost.com/2014/04/17/how-prescription-painkillers-are-killing-us-in-one-chart/.

page 33 "Some fifteen million people worldwide are dependent on opiates" See http://www.who.int/substance_abuse/information-sheet/en/ [accessed March 5, 2016]. This is a 2014 report.

page 33 "around 69,000 people die of opioid overdoses each year" See http://www.who.int/substance_abuse/information-sheet/en/ [accessed March 5, 2016].

page 34 "2.1 million Americans...are currently addicted to legal opioid painkillers" See https://www.drugabuse.gov/about-nida/legislative-activities/testimony-to-congress/2016/americas-addiction-to-opioids-heroin-prescription-drug-abuse.

page 34 "and some 200,000 Canadians" Webster, *CMAJ* 2012, 184(3), pp.285–6.

pages 34–35 "I have been on Tramadol" See https://www.erowid.org/experiences/exp.php?ID=38660 [accessed March 5, 2016].

page 37 "The Opium Eater is bookish" Morrison 2001, p.428.

page 37 "the nervous disposition formerly the privilege of poets" This quote from Thomas Trotter's *A View of the Nervous Temperament* was cited in Dormandy 2012, p.77.

pages 37–38 "Keats's 'Ode on Indolence'" Find the whole 1819 poem here: http://www.poetryfoundation.org/poem/237806.

page 38 "I could not get through the day" Alcott and Nightingale's laudanum use is discussed in Dormandy, 2012, pp.76–84, and Hodgson 2001, pp.68–74. The Florence Nightingale quote appears in an article also by Thomas Dormandy: "Seriously Addictive: A

History of Opium," on the YaleBooks blog by Yale University Press, http://yalebooksblog.co.uk/2012/03/15/seriously-addictive-a-history-of-opium-author-article-by-thomas-dormandy/ [accessed March 5, 2016].

pages 38–39 "The youth with the croaking voice" From *Aretaeus*, an opera written in mid-second century AD, as translated by F. Adams (London 1865) and cited in Dormandy 2012, p.78.

page 39 "eased the tuberculotic sufferings" Dormandy 2012, pp.76–84.

page 39 "John Keats was less fortunate" The disaster of poor Keats's death is discussed in numerous sources, including Dormandy, who describes it as "a horror story" (Dormandy 2012, p.78).

page 40 "Husband run off with a politician?" From Neil Gaiman's 2012 University of the Arts commencement address, which can be found at http://www.uarts.edu/neil-gaiman-keynote-address-2012.

page 42 "First, then, it is not so much affirmed" De Quincey 2013, p.59.

pages 43–44 "Within a minute or so, my attention" Sacks 2012, pp.113–114.

page 46 "the receptors for opioids and endorphins" Stevens, *Bioscience* 2009, pp.1247–1269, available at http://www.ncbi.nlm.nih.gov/pmc/articles/PMC3070387/ [accessed March 5, 2016]. Craig Stevens demonstrates the development of opioid receptors early in vertebrate (not just human) evolution, and then goes further to show that as we evolved, selection pressures seem to have favoured differentiation into different types of opioid receptors with particular pressure toward development in mammals of the euphoria-causing mu-receptor—suggesting that mu-opioid receptors give us a survival advantage. As these receptors and endorphins do very many things in the body, though, this doesn't actually suggest that feeling a high or having addictive tendencies provides a selective advantage. Also interesting is Gavril Pasternak and Ying-Xian Pan's 2013 *Pharmacological Reviews* article, "Mu Opioids and Their Receptors: Evolution of a Concept," which can be found at http://www.ncbi.nlm.nih.gov/pmc/articles/PMC3799236/#B588 [accessed March 5, 2016].

page 47 "a recognized disorder called 'exercise addiction'" Berczik, et al., *Substance Use & Misuse* 2012, available at http://www.ncbi.nlm.nih.gov/pubmed/22216780 [accessed March 4, 2016]. There are other terms for and ways of conceptualizing this phenomenon, and some experiments have challenged the idea that the addictive feeling of a "runner's high" is due to endorphins, e.g., Taylor Hinton's 1986 *Perceptual and Motor Skills* article, "Does placebo response mediate runner's high?", available at http://www.ncbi.nlm.nih.gov/pubmed/3725516.

page 47 "quietly snorted heroin in the bathroom" Blackhurst, *Independent*, April 19, 1997. Available at http://www.independent.co.uk/news/self-admits-taking-heroin-on-pms-jet-1268111.html [accessed March 5, 2016].

pages 47–48 "The surrealist poet Louis Aragon" Self, *The Guardian*, February 1, 2015. Available at http://www.theguardian.com/travel/2015/feb/01/great-city-walks-will-self-take-to-the-streets [accessed March 1, 2016]. Mr. Self has written on the same subject elsewhere and De Quincey often comes up as a key "literary urbanist" and like-minded spirit. He also discusses De Quincey in his 1995 drug-focused collection of essays, *Junk Mail*.

page 48 "A lot of people use walking" McCall, *The Paris Review* 85. Available at http://www.theparisreview.org/interviews/3137/the-art-of-fiction-no-70-malcolm-cowley [accessed February 28, 2016.]

pages 50–51 "If a man 'whose talk is of oxen'" De Quincey (ed. Faflak) 2009, p.54.

page 52 "I was buried for a thousand years" De Quincey (Wordsworth) 1994, p.244.

page 53 "The cursed crocodile" De Quincey (Wordsworth) 1994, p.244.

page 54 "feeling perfectly normal" The guidelines for the 0–10 Pain Scale, via Lucile Packard Children's Hospital Heart Center/CVICU, are explained at https://lane.stanford.edu/portals/cvicu/HCP_Neuro_Tab_4/0-10_Pain_Scale.pdf [accessed March 2, 2016].

page 58 "Marcel Proust began his day with coffee" Burkeman, *The Guardian*, October 5, 2013. Available at http://www.theguardian.com/science/2013/oct/05/daily-rituals-creative-minds-mason-currey [accessed February 16, 2016]. Mind you, while Proust did indeed treat his asthma with various things at various times (including caffeine, morphine, and opium), the smoking powders inhaled as an asthma treatment were probably cigarettes of stramonium, lobelia, and potash, the smoke of which was inhaled as an anti-spasmodic—at least according to Mark Jackson's exhaustive medical study on inhalation of various substances to treat asthma, which can found at http://www.ncbi.nlm.nih.gov/pmc/articles/PMC2844275. I'm not clear if this study means that *The Guardian* is wrong in its idea that Proust took opium powder to treat his asthma at any point.

page 58 "we collectively consumed 6.27 milligrams of morphine per person" From a 2014 International Narcotics Control Board (INCB) report, available at http://www.incb.org/documents/Narcotic-Drugs/Technical-Publications/2014/ND_TR_2014_3_SD_EN.pdf [accessed March 5, 2016]. The 620 tonnes figure provided includes INCB demand estimates for morphine-rich (480 tonnes) and thebaine-rich (140 tonnes) opiate raw materials. Tramadol and other non-controlled opioids are not included in this statistic. These estimates will rise and fall each year and sometimes numbers of one opiate will increase while the supply or demand of another decreases. Generally, the trend seems to be distinctly upward.

page 59 "drugs like tobacco and alcohol are directly associated" Herie and Skinner 2010, p.200.

pages 61–62 "True it is that for nearly ten years" De Quincey (ed. Faflak) 2009, pp.55–56.

page 62 "Quality of life was an invention" Dormandy 2012, p.80. In the introduction to this exhaustive account, Thomas Dormandy slips in his own little confession. As a child, he endured a series of operations eased by an injection before surgery. He writes (pp.3–4): "It transported the present writer into a land of indescribable bliss, never experienced before or since, remembered and cherished between operations long after memories of pain and discomfort had faded. Fortunately he did not realize until many years later that the injection contained a hefty dose of a morphine derivative. Had he known, he would today be an addict or, infinitely more likely, the memory of an addict sadly passed away in his prime. Otherwise his experience has been as a doctor; and he is not animated by any reforming zeal."

page 63 "the spontaneous orgasms one patient experienced" Blaszczak-Boxe, *LiveScience.com*, August 5, 2014. Available at http://www.livescience.com/47208-spontaneous-orgasms-parkinsons-drug-rasagiline.html [Accessed March 3, 2016].

page 64 "according to those in a position to know" See the hydromorphone reports on the online community Erowid (available at http://www.erowid.org/experiences/subs/exp_Hydromorphone.

shtml) for many examples, often both astonishing and evocative. The more research I do, the more I find various substances that are considered to be "closest to heroin" and extremely diverse opinions on the quality of experience of the same drug, even at comparable dosages and levels of opioid tolerance.

page 64 "other patients using it for pain report" See http://www.drugs.com/comments/hydromorphone, for one example. Largely chronic pain sufferers here. It's unclear in most reports whether addiction is an issue, although physical dependence and tolerance clearly are. Regardless, this forum is a repository of experiences of patients who are taking the drugs essentially as prescribed, rather than decidedly recreational users, who may be snorting or injecting equivalent or higher doses of the same prescription medicines, or taking them as suppositories.

page 65 "I tried to drown my sorrows" This is my loose translation of a quote attributed to Frida Kahlo: "Quise ahogar mis penas en el licor, pero las condenadas aprendieron a nadar." There are also various other versions of the phrase, which may be from a 1927 letter. It's unclear if there is a definitive original source, and I have seen various renderings of the phrase in both English and Spanish.

page 66 "I always spent my time painting" This quote is cited in many accounts of Frida's life, for example: http://stmaryriverside.org/school/wp-content/uploads/2012/10/kahlo_additional.pdf.

page 68 "their pain is vastly under-treated or mismanaged" This is a well-documented discrepancy, well described by Judy Foreman in *The Wall Street Journal* (available here: http://www.wsj.com/articles/SB10001424052702304691904579349212319995486). I sense that doctors' treatment of my ankylosing spondylitis—a disease far more common in men— is more respectful and attentive than their treatments of other pain-causing diseases that are more common in women, such as fibromyalgia.

pages 69–70 "Frida Kahlo's life and artwork can serve" Antelo, *Virtual Mentor* 15, May 2013, pp.460–465.

page 71 "Since leaving off opium" De Quincey 1862, p.313.

page 71 "I started out taking a pill" Moondust, a Bluelight.org forum user, writing on March 29, 2014. Available at http://www.bluelight.org/vb/archive/index.php/t-508561.html [accessed January 11, 2016]. There is lots of debate here by recreational prescription drug abusers on whether addiction is inevitable. As "rachamim," another poster on this forum, notes, most participants here will be recreational drug users/addicts: "Taking medicines under medical supervision is an entirely different thing. Very rarely will anyone in this forum be under any kind of supervision." Available at http://www.bluelight.org/vb/threads/345553-tramadol-50mg/page2.

pages 74–75 "Sometimes ah think that people" Welsh 2004, p.8.

page 75 "I trace the origin of my confirmed opium-eating" De Quincey (Wordsworth) 1994, p.24.

page 75 "First Nations communities have declared community emergencies" Webster. *The Lancet* 381, April 27, 2013, pp.1447–1448. Available at http://www.thelancet.com/journals/lancet/article/PIIS0140-6736(13)60913-7/fulltext [accessed March 5, 2016].

page 75 "expressing similar concerns" Dell et al., *Substance Abuse: Research and Treatment* 6, 2012, pp.3–31. Available at http://www.ncbi.nlm.nih.gov/pmc/articles/PMC3411531 [accessed March 4, 2016].

page 76 "In Egypt it has surpassed cannabis" *The Economist*, April 18, 2015. Available at http://www.economist.com/news/middle-east-and-africa/21648690-painkiller-becomes-egypts-favourite-recreational-drug-pill-work-and-play [accessed March 2, 2016]; also, Cunningham, *The Electronic Intifada*, June 30, 2009. Available at https://electronicintifada.net/content/drug-addiction-rise-besieged-gaza/8323 [accessed March 2, 2016].

page 76 "to prevent chemically induced tolerance" McCarthy, *The Guardian*, April 20, 2010. Available at http://www.theguardian.com/world/2010/apr/20/hamas-burns-tramadol-painkillers-smuggled-gaza [accessed March 2, 2016].

page 77 "the bulk of American patients" This was testimony given by Nora D. Volkow, M.D., to the House Committee on Energy and Commerce Subcommittee on Oversight and Investigations on April 29, 2014. Available at https://www.drugabuse.gov/about-nida/legislative-activities/testimony-to-congress/2015/prescription-opioid-heroin-abuse [accessed February 22, 2016].

page 80 "the development of new, powerful opiate analgesics" This has been widely reported. For an example, see Laura Unger's article, "Scientists close in on non-addictive opioid painkillers," in *USA Today*, November 17, 2014. Available at http://www.usatoday.com/story/news/nation/2014/11/17/

non-addictive-opioids-on-horizon/18810059/ [accessed March 1, 2016].

page 81 "yeah there's no way to tell" Bluelight.org forum user nioreho422 writing on June 18, 2010. Available at http://www.bluelight.org/vb/archive/index.php/t-508561.html [accessed February 15, 2016].

page 82 "The habit grew upon him" Sir Arthur Conan Doyle's "The Twisted Lip," in *Sherlock Holmes: The Complete Novels and Stories, Volume 1*, New York: Bantam Books, 1986, pp.308–309.

page 82 "conflates the distinct terms 'dependency' and 'addiction'" For example, in the American Academy of Neurology's position paper taking the first major stand against long-term prescription of opioids for non-cancer pain, dependence, addiction, and overdose are all lumped together—although dependence, like tolerance, is an expected outcome of long-term use. The World Health Organization likewise often uses the terms "addiction" and "dependence" interchangeably. Dependence requiring tapering to avoid withdrawal symptoms is common with other medicines, including SSRI and SNRI antidepressants, benzodiazepines and tryptophan (used for migraines). For more information, see http://www.who.int/substance_abuse/information-sheet/en and http://www.neurology.org/content/83/14/1277.

page 84 "Cold turkey" refers to the goose-flesh Herrie and Skinner 2010, p.142.

page 84 "kicking the habit" Dormandy 2012, p.199.

page 85 "Horrible! that a man's own chamber" Thomas De Quincey, as cited in Page 1877, p.329.

page 85 "Whatever I may have been writing" Thomas De Quincey in a letter to Mary Russell Mitford, as cited in Morrison 2009, p.366.

page 86 "Margaret attended him through" Morrison 2009, p.198.

page 88 "De Quincey often 'set something on fire'" Morrison 2009, p.359.

page 89 "I hit myself with Nirvana" Dear footnote-reading friends, you are rewarded for your persistence with your very own drugs and pain playlist. Turn down the lights and wallow away.
The Rolling Stones, "Paint it Black"
Terra Naomi, "Vicodin Song"
Neil Young, "Needle and the Damage Done"

The Dandy Warhols, "Not if You Were the Last Junkie on Earth"
Marcy Playground, "Poppies"
Vendetta Red, "Opiate Summer"
Ramones, "Take the Pain Away"
Counting Crows, "Round Here"
Lil Wyte, "Oxy Cotton"
Porter Wagoner and Dolly Parton, "The Pain of Loving You"
Red Hot Chili Peppers, "Under the Bridge"
Stromae, "Rail de Musique "
The Tragically Hip, "Opiated"
The Velvet Underground & Nico, "I'm Waiting for the Man"
The Verve, "The Drugs Don't Work"
James Brown, "King Heroin"
Nine Inch Nails, "Hurt"
Gym Class Heroes, "Pillmatic"
Sarah McLachlan, "Angel"
Green Day, "Give Me Novocaine"
Jimmy Eat World, "Pain"
Jon Foreman, "The Cure for Pain"
Lily Allen, "Everyone's At It"
The La's, "There She Goes"
Blur, "Beetlebum"
Elliot Smith, "Needle In the Hay"
Hector Berlioz, "Symphonie Fantastique"

pages 89–90 "read De Quincey's addiction as part" From Faflak's introduction, De Quincey (ed. Faflak) 2009, p.42.

page 93 "manoeuvres the most intricate" De Quincey (Wordsworth) 1994, p.218.

page 95 "For those few minutes I was living" Arkin, 2011, pp.24–25.

page 99 "Mi pintura lleva con ella" Another possibly apocryphal quote from Frida Kahlo. This one is taken from *Frida & Diego: Quotes* by Maria Tsaneva (Lulu Press, 2013).

page 100 "The drugs she was taking" Burrus 2008, p.102. Translated by Ruth Wilson from *Frida Kahlo: 'Je peins ma réalité'*, Editions Gallimard, 2007.

page 100 "Her body, under the elaborate traditional Tehuana dresses" Description according to Raquel Tiból, cited in Wood, *The Guardian*, May 15, 2005. Available at http://www.theguardian.com/artanddesign/2005/may/15/art2 [accessed January 23, 2016].

page 100 "I hope the leaving will be joyful" From Frida Kahlo's illustrated diary, reproduced at http://www.fridakahlofans.com/LastDiaryEntry.html (English translation mine).

page 101 "her famous, joyous still life of a watermelon" This was generally considered to have been Frida Kahlo's last painting, produced in 1954 and finished days before her death, but it has been suggested, because the quality is much higher than most other work created during this final, heavily medicated period, that it was actually painted in 1952, and the inscription "Viva la vida" was added in 1954, eight days before she died. There is no dispute about *this* date, as she wrote it on the painting herself. See http://www.fridakahlofans.com/co680.html for an image of the painting.

Bibliography

Antelo, Fernando. *Virtual Mentor/AMA Journal of Ethics* 15.5 (2013).

Berczik, K. et al. "Exercise addiction: symptoms, diagnosis, epidemiology, and etiology." *Substance Use & Misuse* 47:4 (2012).

Blackhurst, Chris. "Self admits taking heroin on PM's jet." *The Independent*, April 19, 1997.

Blaszczak-Boxe, Agata. "Woman's Spontaneous Orgasms Triggered by Parkinson's Drug." *LiveScience.com*, August 5, 2014.

Burkeman, Oliver. "Rise and shine: the daily routines of history's most creative minds." *The Guardian Online*, October 5, 2013.

Burrus, Christina. *Frida Kahlo: Painting Her Own Reality*. London: Thames & Hudson, 2008.

Cunningham, Erin. "Drug addiction on the rise in besieged Gaza." *The Electronic Intifada*, June 30, 2009.

De Quincey, Thomas. *Confessions of an English Opium-Eater*, London: Vintage (Random House), 2013.

De Quincey, Thomas. *Confessions of an English Opium-Eater*, Hertfordshire: Wordsworth Editions Limited, 1994.

De Quincey, Thomas. *Historical and Critical Essays Vol. II.* Boston: Ticknor & Fields, 1862.

Dell, et al. "Researching Prescription Drug Misuse among First Nations in Canada: Starting from a Health Promotion Framework." *Substance Abuse: Research and Treatment* 6 (2012).

Dormandy, Thomas. *Opium: Reality's Dark Dream*, New Haven: Yale University Press, 2012.

Duffy, Jonathan. "When heroin was legal." *BBC News Magazine*, January 26, 2006.

Faflak, Joel, ed., *Thomas De Quincey: Confessions of an English Opium-Eater.* PLACE?:Broadview Editions, 2009.

Hayter, Alethea. *Opium and the Romantic Imagination.* London: Faber and Faber, 1968.

Herie, Marilyn, and Wayne Skinner. *Substance Abuse in Canada.* Toronto: Oxford University Press, 2010.

Hodgson, Barbara. *In the Arms of Morpheus.* Vancouver: Greystone Books, 2001.

Macht, David I. "The History of Opium and Some of Its Preparations and Alkaloids." *Journal of the American Medical Association* LXIV.6 (1915).

McCall, John. "Malcolm Cowley, The Art of Fiction No. 70." *The Paris Review* 85:Fall (1982).

McCarthy, Rory. "Hamas burns Tramadol painkillers smuggled into Gaza." *The Guardian*, April 20, 2016.

Morrison, Robert. "Poe's De Quincey, Poe's Dupin." *Essays in Criticism* 51.4 (2001).

Morrison, Robert. *The English Opium-Eater: A biography of Thomas De Quincey*. London: Weidenfeld & Nicolson, 2009.

Page, H.A. *Thomas De Quincey, His Life and Writings: With Unpublished Correspondence*. London: John Hogg & Co, 1877.

Sacks, Oliver. *Hallucinations*. New York: Alfred A. Knopf, 2012.

Sebald, W.G. *Austerlitz*. New York: Modern Library (Random House), 2001.

Self, Will. "Take to the city streets for a walking adventure." *The Guardian Online*, February 1, 2015.

Solnit, Rebecca. *A Field Guide to Getting Lost*. London: Penguin Books, 2005.

Stevens, Craig W. "The evolution of vertebrate opioid receptors." *Frontiers in Bioscience*, January 1, 2009.

Webster, Paul C. "Medically induced opioid addiction reaching alarming levels." *Canadian Medical Association Journal* 184.3 (2012).

Webster, Paul C. "Indigenous Canadians confront prescription opioid misuse." *The Lancet* 381.9876 (2013).

Welsh, Irvine. *Trainspotting*. London: Vintage Books, 2004.

Wood, Gaby. "Anatomy of an icon." *The Guardian*, May 15, 2005.

Acknowledgements

THANK YOU TO all those willing to share their knowledge and perspectives. In particular, thank you to Robert Morrison and Wayne Skinner. Thank you also to David Juurlink and Clifford Woolf. Although this is a book about pain and drugs, it's more importantly also a book about friendship. Thank you to my friends, featured by name (Sonia Singh, Derek Laventure, Emily Gesner) and not. Thank you to Saul Olmos, for Mexico. To Anna Martin and Frederic Kodjayan, for photos. And with greatest love to Edik Zwarenstein, my dad, and Mandy Zwarenstein, my mom and most trusted adviser, for everything. I love you.

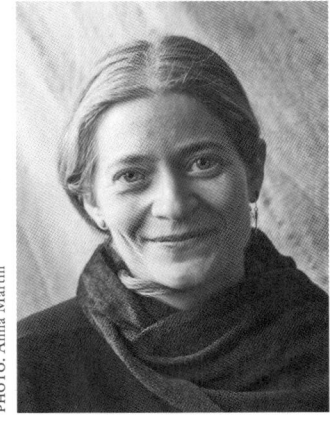

PHOTO: Anna Martin

CARLYN ZWARENSTEIN writes on literature, medicine, social justice, and states of mind. A longtime freelance journalist, she lives in Toronto with her family. This is her first book.
www.carlynzwarenstein.com